WORKING WITH VULNERABLE ADULTS

This text examines the issues of vulnerability in social and health care, exploring the concept of vulnerability and how, welfare services and practitioners may compound or alleviate vulnerability.

Working with Vulnerable Adults develops a sound basis for understanding issues of risk, vulnerability and protection and investigates how agency policies and procedures may, often unintentionally, lead to the voice of service users being marginalised or unheard. Drawing on recent and established research about the protection of vulnerable adults, the book covers:

- Social work, social care settings and vulnerable adults
- The concept of abuse and adult protection
- Using the law in adult protection
- Professional and quality assurance issues
- Assessment and social work with vulnerable adults
- Dealing with and managing vulnerability, risk and abuse
- Adults with mental health difficulties, long-term conditions and learning disabilities
- Community abuse and asylum seekers.

Much contemporary social and health care practice with adults is concerned with issues of risk and protection. *Working with Vulnerable Adults* provides information and knowledge for students and practitioners who are interested in finding out more about this important field.

Bridget Penhale is Reader in Gerontology at the University of Sheffield and Head of Research at the Institute of Health and Social Care Studies, Guernsey, UK.

Jonathan Parker is Professor of Social Work at Bournemouth University, UK.

the social work skills series

published in association with *Community Care*

series editor: Terry Philpot

the social work skills series

- builds practice skills step by step

- places practice in its policy context

- relates practice to relevant research

- provides a secure base for professional development

This new, skills-based series has been developed by Routledge and *Community Care* working together in partnership to meet the changing needs of today's students and practitioners in the broad field of social care. Written by experienced practitioners and teachers with a commitment to passing on their knowledge to the next generation, each text in the series features: *learning objectives; case examples; activities to test knowledge and understanding; summaries of key learning points; key references; suggestions for further reading.*

Also available in the series:

Commissioning and Purchasing
Terry Bamford
Former Chair of the British Association of
Social Workers and Executive Director of
Housing and Social Services, Royal
Borough of Kensington and Chelsea.

Managing Aggression
Ray Braithwaite
Consultant and trainer in managing
aggression at work. Lead trainer and
speaker in the 'No Fear' campaign.

Tackling Social Exclusion
John Pierson
Senior Lecturer at the Institute of Social
Work and Applied Social Studies at the
University of Staffordshire.

Safeguarding Children and Young People
Corinne May-Chahal and Stella Coleman
Professor of Applied Social Science at
Lancaster University.
Senior Lecturer in Social Work at the
University of Central Lancashire.

The Task-Centred Book
Mark Doel and Peter Marsh
Research Professor of Social Work at
Sheffield Hallam University.
Professor of Child and Family Welfare at
the University of Sheffield.

Using Groupwork
Mark Doel
Research Professor of Social Work at
Sheffield Hallam University.

Practising Welfare Rights
Neil Bateman
Author, trainer and consultant specialising
in welfare rights and social policy issues

WORKING WITH VULNERABLE ADULTS

Bridget Penhale and Jonathan Parker

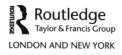

Routledge
Taylor & Francis Group

LONDON AND NEW YORK

communitycare

First published 2008
by Routledge
2 Park Square, Milton Park, Abingdon, Oxon OX14 4RN

Simultaneously published in the USA and Canada
by Routledge
270 Madison Avenue, New York, NY 10016

Routledge is an imprint of the Taylor & Francis Group, an informa business

© 2008 Bridget Penhale and Jonathan Parker

Typeset in Sabon and Futura by
Keystroke, 28 High Street, Tettenhall, Wolverhampton
Printed and bound in Great Britain
by TJ International Ltd, Padstow, Cornwall

British Library Cataloguing in Publication Data
A catalogue record for this book is available from the British Library

Library of Congress Cataloging in Publication Data
A catalog record for this book has been requested

ISBN13: 978–0–415–30190–9 (hbk)
ISBN13: 978–0–415–30191–6 (pbk)
ISBN13: 978–0–203–49293–2 (ebk)

ISBN10: 0–415–30190–4 (hbk)
ISBN10: 0–415–30191–2 (pbk)
ISBN10: 0–203–49293–5 (ebk)

CONTENTS

Case studies   vii
List of illustrations   ix
Acknowledgements   xi

Introduction   1

1   Context and background   7

2   The concept of abuse   22

3   The law   37

4   Performance management, inspection, regulation and quality
    assurance issues   54

5   Assessment   65

6   Vulnerability, risk and abuse   79

7   Mental health difficulties   95

8   Learning disabilities   116

9   Long-term conditions   131

10 Community abuse and asylum seekers   149

    Conclusion   165

    References   172
    Index   183

CASE STUDIES

1.1	Mandy	9
1.2	James	18
1.3	Catherine	19
1.4	Vera	20
2.1	Alan	24
2.2	Henry	32
3.1	Margaret	42
3.2	Oldham Ward	44
4.1	Imran	57
4.2	Building knowledge	63
5.1	Winifred and Edward	74
5.2	Jeremy	77
6.1	Melinda	82
6.2	Tessa	82
6.3	Agnes	86
6.4	Jo	87
7.1	Brenda	96
7.2	Wendy and Tina	109
8.1	James	117
8.2	Local Partnership Board	121
8.3	June	124
8.4	Jim	125
8.5	Sheila	128
9.1	Emily	132
9.2	Daisy	140
9.3	Diana	142
9.4	Joan	143
9.5	Robert	144
10.1	George	153
10.2	Ahmed	162
10.3	Anti-terror legislation and communities	162
10.4	Traveller community	163

ILLUSTRATIONS

BOXES

1.1	Vulnerability and the code of practice for social care workers	11
2.1	Categories of abuse	27
2.2	Definition of abuse	29
2.3	Causes of abuse in care settings	34
5.1	Assessment questions	72
6.1	Norfolk adult protection policy and procedures	84
7.1	National Service Framework for Mental Health Standards	107
10.1	A brief outline of immigration and asylum seeking in the UK	161

TABLES

2.1	The types and levels of abuse	32
3.1	Legislation and safeguarding adults	38
6.1	Intervention types: abuse by care workers	80
6.2	Intervention types: abuse by relatives	81
7.1	Intervention and mental health	115

FIGURES

2.1	Directions of abuse in care settings	31
2.2	The levels of abuse	31
4.1	The interactions between the three levels of service performance and monitoring	55
4.2	The culture of visibility and accountability in care services	56
6.1	Three interlocking processes of assessment	85
9.1	The levels of partnership	137

10.1   Local and structural drivers for community development   151
10.2   Thompson's PCS interactive model of oppression   155
10.3   Culturagram   164

ACKNOWLEDGEMENTS

There are a number of people without whom this book would not have been possible. The initial concept for the book came from discussion with Terry Philpot, who has remained enthusiastic throughout the process; Kirsty Smy and Grace McInnes of Routledge have been supportive and enduringly patient, allowing time for necessary changes and unforeseen delays.

Thanks are also due to colleagues, many of whom are practitioners, past and present, who stimulate much-needed discussion and creativity in this complex area and who are too numerous to name individually. Heads of Departments have also been supportive to this endeavour. The voices of vulnerable adults with whom we have worked in the past stay with us and sustain our commitment to the issue of abuse and to finding solutions to these complex and sensitive situations.

Our families have experienced disruption and unavailability throughout the production of this book and yet remain steadfast in their support; without them this work could not have been completed. The support which we have derived from each other has maintained our commitment to the issue and to this book. Any errors or omissions are of course our own and are acknowledged as such.

Bridget Penhale and Jonathan Parker

INTRODUCTION

OBJECTIVES

By the end of this chapter you should:

- understand the scope and focus of the book

- be able to place adult protection in context.

RATIONALE

Ever since mum started to lose her memory we've been putting her pension into our account. I mean, it'll come to us in the end, won't it? We're not taking it. We're just worried about her having too much cash in the house and, anyway, she'll never miss it.

(Martha, daughter of Maria who has dementia)

Practitioners in social work and social care are often placed in ethically difficult positions (Hugman, 2005). Despite the increasing emphasis on the involvement of those who use social work and social and health care services, agency policies and procedures may, often unintentionally, lead to the voice of service users being marginalised or unheard (Beresford et al., 2007). Practitioners may have strong beliefs and principles in service user rights but, again without intention, may apply these in a general way that fails to consider specific and individual needs, wants and wishes. Social policies may promote general ideals that ignore the individual, and socially accepted assumptions about age, gender and disability, for example, may contribute to the further exclusion or marginalisation of individuals whose situations, experiences or needs do not match those of the majority. It is ironic that it is those people whose experiences and contexts make hearing their voice fundamental to developing practices who are perhaps most likely to be marginalised. We may sympathise with Martha, perhaps wanting to believe she has her mother's best interests at heart, which she may well do, but we have not heard or attempted to listen to Maria!

In this book, we aim to provide an understanding of current professional practice in social and health care and a practical guide for those working with vulnerable adults, people who have been, are being or are at risk of being abused. As well as examining the ways in which social policy, welfare services and practitioners may compound abuse and vulnerability in social care settings, the book explores a sound basis for understanding issues of risk, vulnerability and protection in relation to vulnerable adults within such settings. We draw on recent and established research concerning what is known about protection and how this relates to working with vulnerable adults. We also need to explore what we mean by vulnerability – itself a contested term – and how this relates to other abuse and harm.

The book comprises two main parts. In the first part of this book (Chapters 1–4), we consider social care as a potential location for abusive situations and working with vulnerability. This necessitates an exploration of key knowledge concerning risk, vulnerability and protection. We introduce historical, developmental and policy frameworks for adult protection and briefly we set the scene to explore in the remainder of the book what social work and social care practitioners with vulnerable adults in these settings might do about such situations.

We need to explore and understand what we mean by contemporary social care settings. In a changing world of health and social care, these settings are likely to continue to evolve, so our definitions will take account of core aspects of care giving that are transferable across agencies, disciplines and settings. These issues are of added importance in relation to the developing context of social and health care owing to policy initiatives such as those contained within government guidance: *No Secrets* (Department of Health, 2000a), the *National Service Framework for Mental Health* (Department of Health, 1999a), the *National Service Framework for Older People* (Department of Health, 2001a) and *Our Health, Our Care, Our Say* (Department of Health, 2006). It is also important given the continuing re-creation and development of social work and social care practice as a result of policy shifts and changes.

The book will be of relevance to contemporary practitioners in social work and allied professions because since the mid-1990s there has been increasing concern about the abuse and protection of adults. The cause has been taken up within the Labour government's modernising agenda, making great demands on services and practitioners to respond to identified needs and meet performance targets. Since October 2001, social services departments have been given lead responsibility for the co-ordination of responses to allegations and situations of abuse. It is clear also that there is a drive towards multi-agency working, integrated teams and inter-professional practice. The first decade of the twenty-first century is a time of great change in service delivery and organisation. Social work and social care practitioners will need to develop effective ways of responding to individuals' and communities' needs, working collaboratively with other professionals and contributing to community and individual safety.

Throughout this text, we aim to provide knowledge of abuse, its development and ways in which it might be tackled across a range of contemporary settings that will also provide transferable approaches and knowledge. We also hope that practitioners will be stimulated to examine social care work and the settings in which it is practised, with a view to improving it and sharing best practice. The book will also be of interest to social and health care students and academics. We hope that the issues raised will also be especially relevant to care givers (family members and friends) and people who use social services. It will establish clear perspectives on the institutional care of vulnerable adults, the abuse that may occur there and ways of addressing such abuse alongside working in a range of community settings.

Throughout the book, where case studies drawn from practice are used, names have been changed in order to preserve anonymity. The scope of the book relates to social work and social care, which in this rapidly changing world necessarily involves work with health care and other professionals in statutory, voluntary and private agencies.

In the first chapter we set out the breadth of activities covered in social work and social care settings. This should not be too controversial for readers who will no doubt be able to locate themselves within the settings, agencies or teams we describe. We also present some context to describe social work today. Social work has been distinguished by its fluid and sometimes rather vague and uncertain nature. Some believe this to be its strength, whilst others opt for a more rigorous, if limiting, approach to definition. In our short debate, we offer some of the key personal and political principles under-pinning the tasks that social workers and social care workers do, without being rigid or prescriptive in definition. We introduce the context for practice in adult protection. Definitions of relevant and key terms such as adult protection, vulnerability and risk are given.

In Chapter 2, we draw together what we know about abuse, vulnerability, the settings in which it occurs and the risk factors associated with abusive situations. Important knowledge is introduced to show the many directions abuse can take and the importance of defining key concepts such as risk, vulnerability and protection. The vexed question of what constitutes abuse is explored and its social construction examined, including the continuing implications for social workers and social care workers involved in adult protection.

We focus on abuse, not only in individual terms but also in respect of the way society and social policies contribute to abusive attitudes, assumptions and service provision. In doing so, this chapter also explores, the uncomfortable area of abusive situations developing and being maintained by staff within social care settings. Recent trends in respect of vulnerable adults are set within recent developments in social policy, changing demography, social context and attitudes. Social work and social services provision to vulnerable adults and in relation to issues concerning safety and protection are considered. This includes examination of the development of care in the community, assessment and care management. Information and analysis concerning service development, legislative and policy issues are also dealt with in this introductory chapter. This includes such initiatives as the government's response to the Royal Commission on Long-Term Care, *No Secrets* and *In Safe Hands*, the White Paper, *Valuing People*, the Care Standards Act, 2000, and the White Paper on adult social and health care, *Our Health, Our Care, Our Say* amongst others.

Chapter 3 shifts the focus to the arena of legislation as it relates to social care and social work practice in care settings. Key elements of legislation and possible implications are introduced. These are explored in the ways in which practitioners are affected by or, indeed, can use these aspects of law and policy to protect people who are, for whatever reasons, vulnerable, exploited or abused. Some of the differences in legislation across the UK are highlighted. Social work and social care practitioners operate within the boundaries of specific legislation, and the agencies in which they work are based on social welfare policies and legislation. Thus some time is spent considering this important contextual material for social work practice.

Chapter 4 ends the first part of the book and seeks to understand the place of quality assurance, inspection, regulation and performance management in contemporary social work and social care, describe key elements of the regulatory process and consider how the processes of monitoring may assist in the protection of adults. Alongside this a critical approach will be taken in which we identify and critique some of the potential drawbacks of performance management, regulation and inspection for person-centred care and adult protection.

The emphasis on accountability, registration and increased 'visibility' of care practices grew rapidly in the last two decades of the twentieth century. The National Health Service and Community Care Act, 1990, and subsequent guidance underscore the importance of monitoring and inspection and the assurance of quality in social and health care as a preferred means of enhancing practice by the regulation of standards. The prominence given to these aspects of provision was continued and given fresh impetus by the 1997 Labour government's modernising agenda that has continued to emphasise service improvement through monitoring and regulation. It is these issues that form the basis of this chapter.

In the second part of the book we consider the ways in which social care practitioners can begin to tackle abuse and manage risk and vulnerability in a range of social work and social care situations. Social and health care practitioners and policy-makers are in central positions to adopt and advance good practice initiatives. From the context and background material explored in earlier chapters, particular work settings and foci are considered. The chapters in the second part of the book directly concern social work and social care practice in adult protection in the contemporary world.

Chapter 5 explores relevant forms of assessment in adult protection work and a review of the care management context for contemporary practice and the single assessment process. Since the key elements of the care management process concern continual assessment and re-evaluation of needs, it is important to provide an appreciation of the strengths and limitations of this mode of practice. However, whilst it is necessary to examine this procedural approach we also need to consider other more empowering, enabling and protective approaches to assessment. Different levels, including community needs and the setting of community care plans and more individualised approaches to the assessment of needs, functional abilities, vulnerability and risk are introduced. Following a discussion of risk, a focus on assessment where matters of safety and protection might be issues will develop. A range of strategies is explored in respect of their availability, effectiveness and the resources needed to ensure they are in place. We look at the levels at which abuse occurs and examine social policies and legislation, agency procedure and practice as well as individual techniques of intervention in tackling abuse and managing risk.

The sixth chapter takes a multi-level and multi-dimensional approach to working effectively to reduce and counter abuse. In essence, this means that we consider legislation and social policy issues which are relevant to developing positive long-term strategies to counteract abuse wherever this occurs (either in the domestic arena or in care settings). There is a consideration of local and regional policy initiatives, procedural issues developed across organisations, agencies and within teams. Within this discussion, the importance of partnership and multidisciplinary working between the different agencies involved is emphasised. The limitations of care management approaches and the centrality of risk assessment or risk management approaches are critiqued.

Chapters 5 and 6 form a general practice backdrop to subsequent discussions and include a debate and acknowledgement of moves toward partnerships, collaboration and working with others to protect and meet needs effectively.

It is recognised that some vulnerable adults are likely to experience a range of mental health problems and may be in need of protection. In Chapter 7 we explore some of the potential challenges this presents to practitioners and to policy-makers. Concerns about risks, vulnerability and the need for protection for vulnerable adults and others add complexity to the debate and form much of the discussion relating to the reforms of mental health legislation. The chapter examines contemporary practice with people with mental health problems, as well as some of the risks and needs for protection, including protection from abuse, of people experiencing mental illness. The chapter also considers the needs of informal carers such as family members and friends, and looks at some of the ethical dilemmas that can arise in working in this field.

Chapter 8 concerns the protection of adults with learning disabilities. We consider contemporary social work and social care services for adults with learning disabilities who are deemed vulnerable or in need of protection, together with an examination of risk, vulnerability, protection and abuse and some of the ways in which social workers might respond to such issues. We also look at the particular needs of informal carers as well as people with learning disabilities themselves. This includes an exploration of some of the ethical issues relating to capacity and the right to take risks.

The needs of people experiencing long-term conditions are examined in Chapter 9. This includes individuals with physical disabilities and sensory impairments as well as people who have long-term, or even life-limiting, illnesses that are predominantly physical in origin. As in the previous two chapters, we look at social care and social work services in relation to service users with such conditions before moving to consider and explore issues relating to mistreatment and protection. We also explore the needs of carers who are providing care for individuals with long-term conditions.

Chapter 10 looks at the awareness of abuse as an issue that is wider than concerns affecting people at an individual level and considers community-level abuse especially in respect of asylum seekers and refugees. This chapter examines the uses of community aspects of social work within the contemporary contexts of health and social care and the role of this in working with asylum seekers and other disadvantaged groups to prevent and challenge abuse, discrimination and marginalisation. As well as dealing with anti-oppressive and anti-discriminatory approaches to social care practice in an overarching way, we consider here ways in which social care workers can work alongside asylum seekers and communities to combat community abuse.

In the concluding section of the book we draw together the implications of our exploration and suggest some ways forward in improving the quality and effectiveness of responses to the abuse of vulnerable adults, considering training, supervision and support needs of staff, management processes and social support.

ABOUT THE ACTIVITIES, CASE STUDIES AND BOXES

Each chapter includes a section recommending additional reading. A summary is provided at the conclusion of each chapter. Case studies are used as appropriate, and activities are introduced that allow readers to put knowledge into practice contexts. This will assist the reader by promoting communication of key ideas, thus making it more accessible for adult learners, practitioners undertaking continuing professional development and post-qualifying awards as well as those who are studying for a qualification in social work or social care.

CHAPTER 1

CONTEXT AND BACKGROUND

OBJECTIVES

By the end of this chapter you should:

- understand the role of a social care practitioner with vulnerable adults

- be able to describe some of the key elements of social care and social work

- be able to describe some of the particular settings in which social care takes place

- be able to discuss the different service user groups that comprise adult social care and their possible needs for protection.

INTRODUCTION

In this chapter we consider the range of care settings and the changing world of social work and social care within them. The tasks and roles of practitioners in these settings are introduced, as are the various service user groups with whom social workers and social care workers come into contact during their practice. The dynamic but sometimes fraught question 'what is social work?' is addressed first in order to set the context for the chapter.

UNDERSTANDING SOCIAL WORK TODAY

ACTIVITY 1.1

Spend a few minutes thinking about what you understand as social work. Write down three or four key themes, roles or activities that you might associate with social work and bear these in mind as you read through the rest of this chapter.

It may help you to read Payne (2005) if you are particularly interested in the historical development of social work in the UK and to read the introductory book by Horner (2006) concerning what is social work.

If you ask a member of the public to tell you what social workers do or to tell you what social services can offer, you may get a range of responses largely based on media stories, which are usually negative, or anecdotes based on personal experiences. In the main, it is likely that you will hear either about alleged failings of the child protection system or scare stories relating to potentially dangerous people who are mentally ill. Indeed, if you consider the recent development of social policy it is littered with references to dangerousness and control, seeking to make individuals vulnerable whilst containing vulnerability. Alternatively, more personal good and bad experiences about relatives who have had some contact with a social worker or in residential care may be mentioned. However, for those working in social work and social care or indeed using the services, the story is much more complex. The range of settings and agencies has grown, and the roles and tasks of practitioners within them have increased in recent years. This has become much more complex as a result of the government's modernising agenda for social care, which has been taking place over the last two decades.

Since the full implementation of the National Health Service and Community Care Act, 1990, in April 1993 in England and Wales, social care settings have widened to include providers of social care from local authorities, voluntary agencies and private organisations. Whilst there has always been a mixed economy of social care, the increased emphasis on choice and consumerism has changed the very concept of social work and social care. The tasks associated with community care assessments, the planning, implementing and reviewing process of care management, have further redefined social work and social care. Postle's work shows how perceptions of practitioners about their role and tasks have changed more than practice, however (Postle, 2002).

Perhaps the most obvious change has been the separation, in many Councils with Social Services Responsibilities (CSSRs), which is the new name for what were known as Social Services Departments or authorities, of commissioning services, which remain legally the responsibility of the local authority, and the provision of services, which can be bought in from this expanding range of agencies and organisations. This means, for example, that whereas previously a person could obtain help at home from a Home Care service organised and run by the council, this type of help is now likely to be provided by a privately run care agency, although the CSSR may well retain responsibility for arranging this, so that the individual makes payments for or towards the cost of the care to the CSSR rather than to the agency direct.

The modernisation changes we have just discussed do not just affect social care services, however, as we have also seen changes in the world of health care in recent years. The changing role of health providers, the development of Primary Care Trusts and within them Primary Care Teams, and the increasing emphasis on community and social aspects of nursing and health professionals such as occupational therapists, has led to a blurring of social and health care provision. Whilst this may be confusing, even threatening at times, for practitioners from particular disciplines, it is perhaps the role and tasks undertaken that are of greater importance to service users than the name or indeed the qualification of the person providing the service.

CASE STUDY 1.1: MANDY

Mandy worked as an unqualified co-ordinator of adult care before taking her DipSW (the Diploma in Social Work qualification) in the mid-1990s. After qualifying in 1996, she returned to her area team as a care manager with responsibility for undertaking community care assessments for adults and developing Care Plans to meet identified and agreed needs. The role was familiar to her but the team had undergone a number of changes that were at first disconcerting. Her team manager was now Jane, an occupational therapist from a hospital background, with whom she had collaborated previously when co-ordinating care for people being discharged form hospital. There were two other qualified care managers in the team: one was a social worker like herself and the other was a nurse by profession. Some of the service users that Mandy had worked with prior to training still received assistance and a service from the team. Mandy was reassured to note that the service users were concerned not with the professional background of the practitioners but whether services that were provided following the assessments were appropriate or adequate to meet their individual needs.

It is important to note that whilst blurring professional roles and boundaries can be somewhat disturbing for practitioners, especially initially, service users remain the central focus of social care, and the impact of such organisational changes may not be as great as practitioners fear at the beginning. It is quite likely that the service user may not mind what the professional background of the practitioner is as long as they are effective and efficient and professional in both their practice and their manner. As such it is the values that underpin social work and social care that must be referred to when suspicions or uncertainties for practitioners may work to confound good practice.

At present, the ways in which services are delivered and organised are again undergoing changes. This has pretty much been the case since the change of government in 1997. The modernising agenda in social care effectively began with the publication of the government White Paper in 1998 (see further in Chapter 4). This paper emphasised the importance of promoting independence for vulnerable people, of working together across professions and of closer links between social and health care for adults who need services. The need for greater consumer choice and accountability as well as a clear emphasis on improving effective protection of service users who are at risk was highlighted. These principles were enshrined in the Health Act, 1999, and have been further strengthened by legislation such as the Care Standards Act, 2000, as we will see later, in Chapter 3.

The National Care Standards Commission was set up under the Care Standards Act, 2000, to ensure that services were regulated and that clear and consistent standards were established. It has been taken forward by the creation of an integrated service comprising the Commission and the Social Services Inspectorate (formerly part of the Department of Health), and is now known as the Commission for Social Care Inspection (CSCI). Further changes are anticipated in 2008 when CSCI will merge with the Commission for Health Improvement and the Mental Health Act Commission. The National Service Frameworks for mental health, older people and the White Paper, *Valuing People* (Department of Health, 2001a), concerning learning disability, are adding to the development of services that operate more closely with health care professionals and health systems. These changes are driving the need to reconceptualise social work and social care and once again to promote these areas as distinctive and important agencies in making a difference in people's lives.

At the same time that these developments are transforming the landscape of social work and social care, however, comparable changes are taking place in respect of expectations of qualified social workers. Social work has traditionally been notoriously difficult to define and has laboured under many misconceptions, public and otherwise. Latterly, there has been growing acceptance and adoption of the following definition of social work agreed by the International Association of Schools of Social Work and International Federation of Social Workers in 2001:

> The social work profession promotes social change, problem solving in human relationships and the empowerment and liberation of people to enhance well-being. Utilising theories of human behaviour and social systems, social work intervenes at the points where people interact with their environments. Principles of human rights and social justice are fundamental to social work.

This definition provides a much more positive view of social work and reclaims its aim to effect change, to empower and enable individuals whilst also focusing on social, structural and political factors affecting people. It advances the more common individually focused definitions (see Thomas and Pierson, 2006). The definition also promotes the use of knowledge, theories and models to enhance effective practice and roots itself in the values of social justice and human rights.

This definition has been taken up within the National Occupational Standards for Social Work and is seen as something to which social workers can and should subscribe. The Standards bring with them a set of core values for social work and social workers that concern the need for good interpersonal skills and information sharing, being service-user-led, able to advocate on behalf of others and to work openly with other professionals from different disciplines. These key values concern respect for individuals, families, carers, groups and communities, honesty about role and resources, commitment to empowerment and ability to challenge discrimination. These are associated with the General Social Care Council's (GSCC) Codes of Practice for Social Care practitioners and agencies, which have been produced. There is an opportunity for social work to assert its position in working to protect vulnerable people at an individual, policy or agency and social structural level. Social work's location at the intersection between society and those excluded from it in some way is confirmed within this.

We must acknowledge here that not everyone working within social care settings is a social worker. However, the Codes of Practice which have been developed by the GSCC set forth certain expectations and standards, which are common to all involved in social care, including employers (GSCC, 2002). Social care practitioners must safeguard the rights of individuals as far as possible, maintaining public trust and working to increase choice whilst balancing rights and risks. The emphasis in the GSCC Code of Practice for Social Care Workers is on probity and on protecting service users who are in some way vulnerable: some examples are shown in Box 1.1.

BOX 1.1 VULNERABILITY AND THE CODE OF PRACTICE FOR SOCIAL CARE WORKERS

As a social care worker you must respect the independence of service users and protect them, as far as possible, from danger or harm. This includes:

- challenging dangerous, abusive, discriminatory or exploitative behaviour and using established processes and procedures to report it
- taking complaints seriously and responding to them or passing them to the appropriate person
- respecting confidential information and gaining permission from those it concerns to share it for specific reasons e.g. consultation with managers or other members of the care team
- recognising the potential for power imbalances in working relationships with service users and carers and using authority in a responsible manner
- following practice and procedures designed to keep you and other people safe from violent and abusive behaviour at work.

As a social care worker you must, to the best of your ability, balance the rights of service users and carers with the interests of society. This includes:

- taking necessary steps to prevent service users from doing actual or potential harm to themselves or other people.
- balancing the rights of service users whose behaviour represents a risk to themselves or other people with the paramount interest of public safety.

Other aspects of the Code of Practice concern the importance of maintaining a professional focus, of keeping up to date in terms of knowledge and skills and of consultation if circumstances change which may make practitioners less able to complete their role. The centrality of good practice and not abusing, harming or exploiting service users in any way is stressed. The Code promotes anti-discriminatory practice as a key element here.

However, it is not just social workers and social care staff who are subject to a Code of Practice. The second Code of Practice produced by GSCC sets out its expectations for employers. The details of this Code are also relevant to work with vulnerable adults and abusive situations. The importance of ensuring that social care practitioners are suitable to work with people in care settings is highlighted. This includes completing various checks but also refers to supporting the continuing training and development of staff in order to meet service users' needs and also to ensure that practice is safe.

ACTIVITY 1.2

Consult the GSCC website and compare the two elements of the Code of Practice – one for employees and one for employers (www.gscc.org.uk). Identify those aspects of the Code of Practice for Employers that could have an impact on the protection of vulnerable adults and consider these in the light of the Code of Practice for Employees. What are the similarities and implications for practice?

Importantly, the Codes recognise that social care practitioners may act abusively. Unfortunately, they do not explicitly acknowledge that social care workers may themselves experience abuse or be abused by other individuals, including service users, their agency or the roles and tasks prescribed to them. This is something admirably dealt with by Jack (1994), who argues convincingly that many of the workers who are marginalised and excluded in terms of pay and conditions, and who are often women, work with the most vulnerable and excluded people within care settings. Jack argues further that the power differentials within such settings may lead to abusive situations arising.

As we will see in Chapter 3, legislation has been implemented from 2004 (under the Care Standards Act, 2000) to establish the Protection of Vulnerable Adults list, which effectively acts as a workforce ban. The GSCC Code of Practice for employers identifies the necessity for ensuring that unsafe practitioners are not employed but fails to emphasise the importance of employing agencies in setting up non-abusive settings that value staff. As Kitwood (1997) noted in respect of dementia care, valuing staff is central to preventing poor social and emotional care. The evidence for the promotion of good practice is seen in the creation of specialist residential facilities for people with dementia (Dean et al., 1993; Lindesay et al., 1991).

The British Association of Social Workers has recently produced a welcome revision of its Code of Ethics (BASW, 2002). This Code, again, relates directly to the role of social workers in working to protect and empower people who are vulnerable, and to prevent abuse. The BASW Code identifies five basic social work values:

- human dignity and worth
- social justice
- service to humanity
- integrity
- competence.

These principles are helpful in promoting social justice as well as individual service. When working with abuse, it is clear that social and political structures have the potential to abuse or create conditions in which abuse is more likely to occur. Social workers in care settings are to be encouraged not only to work towards preventing and reducing individual abuse but to identify and highlight practices and policies that contribute to the potential abuse of service users.

UNDERSTANDING CARE SETTINGS

Although in this book we mainly talk about care settings, when considering definitions and terminology we also need to look briefly at what we understand by the term 'institution'. As with abuse, there is no standard definition of an institution. Dictionary definitions provide a number of different meanings for the word. Institution may mean a society or organisation. The word concerns structure, function and process, not merely the presence of a physical entity or building (Jack, 1998). In a reconsideration of residential provision, Jack suggests that the term 'institution' has become synonymous with a particular form of service provision and processes of institutionalisation (Jack, 1998). He argues that a somewhat simplistic, dualistic concept can be identified within both public and professional arenas and suggests that this concept equates community with good features and institutions with all that is bad. Whilst Jack is surely correct to challenge such oversimplifications, his alternative model, which contrasts neglect in the community with high-quality residential care, appears equally misleading. It is notable, also, that his analysis fails to include any detailed consideration of institutional abuse (see Chapter 2 for further discussion of this).

For the purposes of this book, 'institution' refers to care provided within an environment which is not owned by the individual, and where the locus of control lies beyond the individual living in that environment. Also central to the definition is that the individual lives with others and there is likely to be little, often no, choice as to who those individuals are. Control over the structure, function and organisation of the home is not within the power of the individual but is owned by members of staff who are not ordinarily resident in that environment. Indeed, the extent of control, or lack of control, and agency by individuals in relation to their living environment appears to be a key defining element of an institution although the degree of control available to them is likely to vary between different settings.

However, those in institutional care settings may find their care and control limited and may experience themselves as situated anywhere on a long continuum stretching from choice to coercion. It is widely assumed, in these days of post-community care provision, that the majority of adults who live in residential care are there by choice. This is in stark contrast to those who are in prison, or those individuals who are committed to psychiatric or Special Hospitals under the provisions of the Mental Health Act, 1983.

Similarly, some older people may still experience a lack of real choice when faced with the ways that local authorities act in assessing their needs and the use of a number of rationing devices by them. Authorities may talk about providing increased choice for individuals, yet provide such strict eligibility criteria, particularly in relation to service provision once needs have been assessed, that the individual experiences limited or false choice. Entry into residential or perhaps more frequently nursing home care may often occur through lack of realistic and (economically) viable alternatives for the individual to remain in the environment of their choice. Such initiatives as the National Service Frameworks for Mental Health and for Older People and *Fair Access to Care* (Department of Health, 2003a), although they have the potential to assist with this, do not appear to have provided solutions up until now.

Much of the care within institutional settings is valuable, of good quality and well provided. In many recent statements about institutional care there seems to be a polarisation between community living as first choice and institutional care pretty much as a last resort. This has not been helped by many of the statements surrounding the implementation of the community care reforms which appeared to imply that community provision is the only appropriate form of care which is relevant for individuals. However, whilst avoiding the oversimplified conflict model of community care versus institutions, we must not ignore the testimonies of service users in general, and of survivors of institutional abuse in particular (Stanley et al., 1999). Such testimonies tend to affirm a view that care in community settings is more desirable for individuals than continuing long-term care in institutions, particularly if those settings are ones in which abuse occurs and in some instances is perpetuated.

Power relations are central to all abusive situations. What need to be considered are the dynamics and variables which inform the abuse of power within different settings. The work of Goffman provides a vivid backdrop against which any exploration of the working of power within care settings takes place (Goffman, 1961) and it is helpful briefly to introduce some key ideas at this point.

In the early 1960s, Goffman published his seminal work on institutions (Goffman, 1961). In this influential text he constructed a model of the 'total institution' and explored the processes of depersonalisation which individuals experience through living in such institutions. Goffman looked at the routines and structures of institutions. Within his work he identified five basic types of institutions. These were:

- institutions designed to care for the 'incapable and harmless' (e.g. homes for the 'blind, aged or orphaned')
- institutions established to care for the 'incapable' who present an unintended threat to the community (e.g. sanatoriums; mental hospitals)
- institutions organised to protect the community from 'intentional dangers' (e.g. prisons)
- institutions established for some 'worklike task' (e.g. army barracks; boarding schools)
- institutions set up as retreats from the world (e.g. monasteries).

It is with the first two types we are mainly concerned in this book. The key area of institutional provision not covered here is that of penal institutions. We decided to concentrate on settings that provide care, protection and sometimes treatment for individuals. In these places, the duty of care is perhaps of paramount concern, and, when abuse occurs in such settings, it may thus be perceived as more especially at odds with the institution's stated function. In penal settings such as prisons, definitions of abuse need to be constructed in the context of rather different institutional objectives such as crime prevention and punishment and, within such institutions, care perhaps becomes of somewhat lesser concern.

For Goffman, all these different types of institutions shared some common characteristics, albeit to varying degrees. According to Goffman, the key features of total institutions were:

> First all aspects of life are conducted in the same place, and under the same single authority. Second, each phase of the members' daily activity is carried on in the immediate company of a large batch of others, all of whom are treated alike and required to do the same thing together. Third, all phases of the day's activities are tightly scheduled with one activity leading at a pre-arranged time into the next, the whole sequence of activities being imposed from above by a system of explicit formal rulings and a body of officials.
>
> (Goffman, 1961, p. 17)

In Goffman's view, it was the basic nature of institutions and care provided within these settings, which lead to a degradation of that care. Goffman argued that the removal of normal, everyday patterns of activity and identities for individuals provided a specific cultural and social context for institutional care. It was within those specific contexts for particular institutions that individuals became depersonalised (Goffman, 1961). And it is within this context of depersonalisation that abuse may occur. As Wardhaugh and Wilding suggest when looking at the corruption of care, if we start from a perspective in which individuals are viewed as in some way less than human and 'not like us', then abuse of those individuals becomes more understandable, if not justifiable (Wardhaugh and Wilding, 1993). Through a process of 'othering', those people who are excluded and determined as the 'other' are more likely to be marginalised and to experience abuse as a consequence.

ACTIVITY 1.3

Think of an institution that you are familiar with (such as a school, college or care service) and compare it with Goffman's critique. Identify where you think there are similarities and differences with the analysis and highlight how this might impact on those living within it.

In recent years there has been some criticism of Goffman's work, arguing that his account did not really examine the relationship between the institution and the broader social context in which care was provided (Perring, 1992). Moreover, few current institutions now fit neatly within Goffman's original definition. For example, not all aspects of life are carried out in one place (young people who are accommodated in care homes attend school; occupation or training outside of the establishment may be provided for adults who live in care homes); not all activities are carried out by all individuals at the same time, nor are all aspects of the regime rigidly programmed at all times. However, his analysis of institutional life still has relevance today and an understanding of this is needed if we are to adequately consider abuse in care.

THE CHANGING CONTEXT OF CARE

In examining abuse in care settings, it is necessary to recognise the changing nature of care settings and the care provided by them. These recent changes form part of the structural changes in welfare provision in the United Kingdom, which have taken place over the past twenty-five years or so.

The 1960s and 1970s witnessed the growth of the movement towards community care and the provision of care to individuals in their own homes. As we have seen in the last section, this was coupled with the development of views concerning the detrimental effects of institutional life and 'batch living' on individuals. The combination of these two elements resulted in the concept of care in the community with associated changes in social policy taking place to secure the changes needed for community care to become a reality in the early 1990s. These policy changes took place together with legislative change in the form of the National Health Service and Community Care Act, 1990, which was finally fully implemented in 1993. This framework has seen the further development of perceptions of institutions as places of last resort for individuals and the range and scope of institutional care and care settings has been altered as a consequence.

In recent decades, owing to the implementation of community care policies, there has been an overall decrease in the number of institutions in the public sector and a rise in the number of institutions for adults which are run by the private or not-for-profit (including the voluntary) sector (Peace et al., 1997). We have witnessed the closure of a large number of children's homes and of traditional psychiatric hospitals. Institutions are generally smaller in size and more diverse in terms of their provision: for example the amount of respite care provision for shorter, temporary periods of time has increased (Moriarty and Levin, 1998). They are less likely to be isolated, and many residential homes are now more integrated into the communities in which they are located.

There has also been a rise in the number of small residential homes offering care to a very small number of residents who may in some instances actually be considered as part of a family (Peace and Holland, 1998). Nevertheless, these remain institutions in as much as there is an organisational setting in which care is provided and finance is exchanged in relation to the provision of care. As we shall see in the next chapter, matters of the registration, inspection and regulation of care homes within the legislative framework of the Registered Homes Act, 1984, are also of relevance here concerning these organisational settings and the basis on which they are established and operate.

In relation to the contractual basis of care provided within residential (and nursing home) care settings, the tenure of the individuals who live within them is also significant in this context. Central to such considerations are the role and nature of the care contract between the institution and the service user. This has both explicit and implicit elements. It may, of course, be less explicit for some groups than others: for example, children and mental health service users may not be signatories to a contract. However, within the field of learning disabilities and in the care of older people, contractual arrangements are much more likely to be used. This is especially evident in relation to those individuals who are in receipt of assistance via public funding for their care, when the contract is likely to include the local authority as a party. It may be the case that the formal contract that is established in such instances is essentially between the local authority and the provider (the institution) rather than with the individual who receives the care. In these instances too it is possible that the individual service user is not a signatory to the contract in any formal sense.

What is often found are rather more implicit, perhaps more informal contracts between the individual service user and the provider and between the local authority or health purchaser and the individual. It is possible to consider this contract as being triangular in form: between the service user, the provider (institution) and the state (as purchaser and regulator of care). Such contracts, whether implicit or explicit, charge the institution with a duty of care with regard to individuals who are vulnerable. The existence of abuse within such settings can be viewed as a failure to ensure that the duty of care is upheld and can be conceptualised as a violation of the implicit terms of the contract.

CARE SETTINGS

However, in this book we are not just looking at care settings where people live. There are many different care settings that we can identify. These include, but are not exhausted by, the following:

- hospitals
- hospices
- nursing homes
- residential care
- Primary Care Teams (PCTs)
- resource or day centres and day hospitals
- voluntary or community lunch clubs and specifically focused groups.

The Care Standards Act, 2000, provides a definition of 'care homes', which is helpful to our understanding of care settings. This is as follows:

> S.3 – (1) For the purposes of this Act, an establishment is a care home if it provides accommodation, together with nursing or personal care, for any of the following persons.
>
> (2) They are –
>
>   (a) persons who are or have been ill;
>   (b) persons who have or have had a mental disorder;
>   (c) persons who are disabled or infirm;
>   (d) persons who are or have been dependent on alcohol or drugs.
>
> (3) But an establishment is not a care home if it is –
>
>   (a) a hospital;
>   (b) an independent clinic; or
>   (c) a children's home,
>   or if it is of a description excepted by regulations.

A discussion of how social workers are likely to be involved in these settings, and what their tasks and roles might be, is helpful at this point. Changes in the world of social and health care have meant that there has been an increasing blurring of roles and tasks, as we have seen above. However, practitioners in social care settings are providing services to assess needs, to plan and organise care services, to liaise with other professionals and co-ordinate the provision of services, to act as a focal point for service users and carers and to review services that have been provided. Also, social care practitioners may well be providing services directly to service users or carers. They may undertake personal care, assist with activities of daily living and act as an advocate in everyday tasks and situations. Practitioners in social care settings will complete a range of these tasks outlined. This is shown in the following case study.

CASE STUDY 1.2: JAMES

James Dodgson worked as a social worker completing community care assessments of people prior to discharge from hospital. In his assessment of Marie Overton, a forty-five-year-old woman with advanced ovarian cancer, it was identified that she wished to talk through the implications of her illness, her regrets in life and what would happen to her children when she died. James was not in a position to offer such work, neither was he the most appropriate person to take on the task as he was not trained in the specialist area of palliative care. He was aware that she wished to return home for her care and did not wish to enter the local hospice if possible. However, James negotiated with her for the hospice social worker, Jill, to see her and offer her space to talk through issues.

At a later date, when more care was needed, James and Jill helped Marie to negotiate an increase in social care assistance at home as well as nursing care, which helped her to remain at home.

The roles of James, Jill and the social care workers were different but fulfilled many of the roles and tasks outlined above.

SERVICE USER GROUPS AND SOCIAL CARE

Care services are offered by statutory, voluntary and private providers. This has always been the case, but is perhaps more recognised nowadays. The adult populations for whom care services are provided are equally diverse. However, what is common to all services is that they work with some of the most vulnerable and/or marginalised people within society. The following groups of people are likely to be included as service user groups in adult care settings:

* people with learning disabilities
* people with mental health problems

- people with physical, including sensory, disabilities
- people who are homeless
- people with life-threatening illnesses or other major health conditions
- people unable to live on their own
- people with substance misuse difficulties
- people who are meeting socially.

It is important to note that older people who are disadvantaged and vulnerable may be included within the groups listed above. Social workers may be involved with individuals from any of these groups. They may work generically, across the range of adult service users, or they may work specifically with one group as a specialist worker in that area. Social care workers, on the other hand, are likely to be working in a particular specialism in terms of service users. Since the implementation of the community care reforms in the early 1990s, we have seen the gradual development of social care work with adult service users.

It is perhaps almost a cliché, but important none the less, that, for whatever reasons a person becomes a service user, they are and remain a person first and foremost. At a time when an individual's personhood may be challenged or they become vulnerable because friends and relatives, the wider community and care services may see an illness or label rather than the individual behind it, it goes without saying that social care practitioners promote a 'person-first' approach. This is aided by using such phraseology as 'people with . . .' rather than an all-encompassing and homogenising adjective such as 'the dying' or 'the elderly'. The latter terms suggest that all people within that particular group share the same experiences, outlook and future experiences and are part of the same undifferentiated group. Such an approach denies their individuality; the former approach promotes the person. The following case study demonstrates this.

CASE STUDY 1.3: CATHERINE

Catherine Upton had worked at the Greenlands Day Centre for six months. It was a centre that catered for a range of members with different needs. Thursdays were allocated for people with dementia. She had become increasingly concerned about fellow care workers who complained about 'the demented' who ought, in some of her colleagues' opinions, to be 'put away because they weren't really people any more'. Catherine had recently attended a training course in which person-centred care featured highly. She attempted to treat all members as individuals and asked carers and relatives for personal details in order to help her to plan the way she would respond to individual members. One relative, the daughter of an eighty-three-year-old man, commented that she had forgotten her father was 'a real person with his experiences, needs and wishes' until Catherine had asked these details and had spoken to her not about 'the demented' but the person her father was. Catherine decided to raise the issue of language and discussed with her manager how this might best be done. It was decided that one of the regular staff meetings should be used for staff members to look at this issue.

It is important that social work, social care and health care practitioners do not inadvertently worsen abuse because of the complexity of social and health care agencies, by not clearly explaining their roles or by working independently from other professions who are also involved with a particular service user. The following case study describes, unfortunately, a situation that is not uncommon.

CASE STUDY 1.4: VERA

Vera Sutcliffe and her husband, Jim, had been married for thirty-five years. Jim was an amateur boxer in his youth and was his regiment's champion when on National Service in Malaysia. He gave up when he married Vera and worked as a driver for a local haulage company. Over the last five years Jim had had two strokes that left him with a permanent weakness on his left-hand side and an intermittent frustration that on occasions led to violent outbursts. He had threatened to hit Vera and once manhandled the insurance man from the house.

Vera and Jim were worried by these changes and asked their General Practitioner, Dr Kapur, for some help. Dr Kapur said he would refer Jim to the Community Psychiatric Nurse, who he said would be able to 'sort things out for her'. Vera thought that this might give her a break from Jim when tired or when he was becoming frustrated. She was unsure whether she would get help with the practical aspects of caring for Jim, but thought she would ask when the nurse came.

When the CPN visited, she took full details of the situation, but did not feel she could offer anything at the present time. She suggested that Vera might like some help from social services. Vera was confused because she had not thought social services were any different from the nurse. However, she agreed to the CPN passing on details. When the social worker came she took all the same details that the CPN had taken. When Vera asked directly what practical help and advice the social workers could offer and when she could expect it, the social worker said it was not quite so simple as she needed to speak to everyone involved to plan how best to help. She suggested in the meantime that Vera and Jim contact the local Stroke Association.

Vera was upset by the delay, the continued questioning and the passing from one service to another. Jim sensed that Vera was upset and tried to assist her but he quickly became angry, frustrated and lashed out at the social worker. The social worker left the situation quickly and returned to her office. She discussed the case with her manager who decided that Jim was perhaps becoming violent and uncontrollable. He said that no services would be provided if Jim was going to act in a violent, unpredictable and aggressive way and asked the police to visit.

This case study illustrates how situations can quickly become something different to how they originated. The repeated assessments and lack of dialogue between services left Jim and Vera in a difficult and vulnerable situation. Although Jim's difficulties resulted from his stroke, the social work manager saw his frustrations in a different way. The manager withdrew services and saw him as a threat to his staff. Whilst it is not acceptable for social workers to be assaulted, and the manager has a duty to protect his staff, the system failed this couple and made their vulnerability worse.

SUMMARY

In this chapter, we have considered what social work and social care is and the values that underpin it in practice. We have also explored what we mean by care settings and introduced some of the service user groups with whom practitioners are likely to have contact. In the next chapter we explore the meanings of abuse, its development and ways in which it can be understood.

KEY READING

Coulshed, V. and Orme, J. (2006) *Social Work Practice: An Introduction* (4th edition), Basingstoke: Palgrave.

Goffman, E. (1961) *Asylums*, New York: Doubleday.

GSCC (2002) *Codes of Practice for Employees and Employers*, London: General Social Care Council.

Payne, M. (2005) *The Origins of Social Work: Continuity and Change*, Basingstoke: Palgrave.

CHAPTER 2

THE CONCEPT OF ABUSE

OBJECTIVES

By the end of this chapter you should:

▧ understand the different types of abuse that adults may be exposed to

▧ be able to describe some of the key risk factors related to abusive situations

▧ be able to describe some of the particular aspects of abuse in care settings

▧ be able to discuss the different services that might assist adults at risk and in need of protection.

INTRODUCTION

In Chapter 1, we introduced the contexts of social work, social care and social care settings. This chapter discusses the concept of abuse and also the range of potential abusive situations that may occur, including those that may happen in care settings. A typology is outlined in order to ease the identification of different aspects and attributes of abuse. Definitions of risk, vulnerability, abuse and protection are also covered in this chapter, together with a consideration of risk factors for abuse in both domestic and care settings. Perhaps it is with our use of the terms 'vulnerable adults' and 'vulnerability' that some would take issue and so we start with exploring these issues further.

WHO IS VULNERABLE?

It could be argued that every adult is potentially vulnerable in some way or that to refer to someone as vulnerable automatically assigns them a label that would usually be seen in a negative light. It implies an element of weakness, although it does not provide the reason for it. For some people it may be seen to apportion blame for the vulnerability with the vulnerable person. For others the difficulty may be with the likely attribution of 'victim status' to someone referred to as vulnerable. It may be thought that, because of the possible difficulties with it, the term should be avoided and more neutral terms used in respect of the person. The focus should perhaps be on abuse, exploitation and mistreatment by others. This could be seen to remove any suggested blame from the person experiencing the abuse and to place it firmly with the person, people, agency or society responsible for it.

However, we have chosen to continue to use the term 'vulnerable adult' and to refer to 'vulnerability'. In part, this is pragmatic because it is the term that has been commonly used in the UK in relation to the abuse of adults over the past five years and is the term that appears in both legislation and policy guidance. Nevertheless, our use of the term does not mean that we ascribe to blaming the person for their experiences, nor does it mean that we would wish to remove any responsibility from those perpetrating actions that are abusive or any suggestion that the person who experiences abuse should be held responsible for the situation they find themselves in. We would also not see that vulnerability implies weakness in any other way than any of us might be affected by the issues and actions described here given certain situations or conditions. In this book, we use the term 'vulnerable people' to refer to people who, by virtue of their circumstances, and, as a result of the way care services are organised and operated and in the way that wider society treats adults who are differently abled, are placed in a position that makes them vulnerable. In particular this situation is likely to be the case in relation to society in general. Additionally, as we have indicated, it is important to note that the term 'vulnerable adult' is used in the legislation. More specifically, the Care Standards Act, 2000, S.80 (6) defines vulnerable adults as follows:

(a) An adult to whom accommodation and nursing or personal care are provided in a care home.
(b) An adult to whom personal care is provided in their own home under arrangements made by a domiciliary care agency; or
(c) An adult to whom prescribed services are provided by an independent hospital, independent clinic, independent medical agency or National Health Service body.

In this definition there is an important underlying meaning created: services can render a person vulnerable and, as we can see above, vulnerability appears to be viewed largely in relation to service provision. This is important for social care practitioners to bear in mind. We must all be vigilant in ensuring that our practice enables, supports and protects people rather than creating or perpetuating any vulnerability for that person. Additionally, we need to alter practices that serve to make people vulnerable, even if this is unintentional. The following case study demonstrates some of the situations that can arise that may make people vulnerable, or that could act in a way to increase their vulnerability, either in care settings or beyond.

CASE STUDY 2.1: ALAN

Alan Smith was a man for whom independence had been extremely important throughout his life. After experiencing an accident, which left him weakened on his left side and memory-impaired, he was offered day care to help him with personal tasks and to provide a degree of social contact. Alan was pleased by this, but asked that a male worker carry out assistance with personal tasks. He also requested certain types of activities during the course of the day. The manager of the day centre saw Alan and sympathised with his request but explained that he had could not guarantee that a male staff member would be on duty and he would either have to have a female member of staff or not receive assistance. He was also told that, because of staff shortages, they had to put on a 'set menu' of activities and that, unfortunately, he could not simply opt out of activities because of 'health and safety' reasons. Alan therefore decided not to go to the day centre, as they could not meet his needs and seemed to be very much oriented towards services rather than service users. However, Alan's decision not to attend the day centre meant that his needs for social interaction and activities were unmet over a period of time.

The term 'vulnerable adult' is also used in Department of Health guidance. In *No Secrets* (Department of Health, 2000a, 2.3), the term is employed in the same way as it was used in the consultation document relating to mental capacity and decision-making *Who Decides?* (Lord Chancellor's Department, 1998) to describe a person aged over eighteen years:

> who is or may be in need of community care services by reason of mental or other disability, age or illness, and

> who is or may be unable to take care of him or herself, or unable to protect him or herself, against significant harm or exploitation.

It is important to recognise here that 'community care services' refers to more than just those services that we traditionally think of as part of community care. The guidance is clear that in fact, such services also include 'all care services provided in any setting or context' (Department of Health, 2000a, 2.4). Clearly, those services provided at community level by education, leisure or transport departments within local authorities may also be included here.

What is abuse?

Defining what we mean by abuse can also be a rather difficult question. It has exercised the minds of academics, policy-makers and practitioners for many years. For some, it seems that certain hierarchies of abuse have been developed, in which the observable physical acts of mistreatment and assault can appear to be given a higher profile than unseen, emotional and psychological abuse. Others, perhaps, campaign strongly on behalf of a particular group who may be abused in a range of ways, all of which are considered potentially damaging. Such groups may for instance relate to issues of domestic violence, elder abuse or the abuse of people with learning disabilities.

Yet other people may approach the issues from a particular level of action. For instance, for some people, abuse results from individual acts perpetrated by one person against another whilst others may consider organisational policy and practices as responsible for causing abuse. Still other people may believe that abuse results primarily from the way society is organised and structured and the ways in which people are apportioned or even denied their roles, rights and responsibilities. In the case of Alan, in the case study above, it seems clear that nobody was acting in a deliberate way to abuse him or exploit him. However, the care setting in which he was involved increased his vulnerability by not being able to meet his wishes or indeed by placing him in a position in which the care that he needed was evidently not available. This may be construed as abusive in itself.

ACTIVITY 2.1

Take a few minutes to think about situations of abuse that we have mentioned so far. If you were trying to develop a definition of abuse, what aspects would you need to take into account?

Any attempt to gain clarity and agreement on precise and all-encompassing definitions of abuse appear bound to fail for two key reasons. First, it is unlikely that total and full agreement will ever be reached. Vested interests are involved and people usually clarify issues from a particular local and/or cultural level and perspective. For example, it is likely that practitioners, researchers, academics and so forth will all have and use different definitions. This may not matter too much, provided that different groups acknowledge this possibility and are explicit about what definitions they are using and for what purposes (Penhale et al., 2000) and that these are clear for other people to understand, appreciate and work with as necessary. Second, our understanding of what constitutes abuse is constantly changing and developing. It is a fluid concept and is dependent on contemporary notions of acceptable and unacceptable behaviour. To fix our definition of abuse in absolute terms, therefore, could be abusive in itself as, by doing so, we potentially outlaw an individual's experience, if this does not fit with the accepted definition of what behaviour is acceptable as normal. It could also be that those individuals who deal with abuse could fail to identify and act on abuse on the grounds that a particular exact set of criteria is not matched. Such a failure could have disastrous consequences if abuse is not dealt with and resolved.

Indeed, the very notion of abuse is a social construction, one which is created by society and which will therefore be different in different societies. What is viewed as abuse, mistreatment or neglect will therefore vary in time and place; what is seen as abuse at one point in time may not be perceived in this way some years later. Equally, what is accepted as abuse in one society may be quite different in another. We therefore need to bear in mind this important social element, especially when considering responses to violence and abuse and how these vary over time. The focus of the sociological study of social constructionism is to discover the ways in which individuals and groups participate in the creation of their perceived reality. It involves looking at the ways in which social phenomena are created, institutionalised and incorporated into the tradition of that particular society by individuals. Socially constructed reality is seen as an ongoing, dynamic process; reality is produced and re-produced by individuals acting on their interpretations and their knowledge of it. Berger and Luckmann (1966) argued that all knowledge, including the most basic knowledge of everyday reality, is derived from and maintained by social interactions. When people interact, they do so with the understanding that their respective perceptions of reality are related, and, as they act upon this understanding, their common knowledge of reality becomes reinforced.

In view of this social construction of violence, it is probably best to accept that there are many levels at which abuse operates, and that definitions must always remain somewhat fluid and open to constant reinterpretation. If we do not allow for this possibility, we may indeed be abusive ourselves by limiting the person's experience to what we consider appropriate. And as suggested above, this may mean that abuse is not dealt with satisfactorily if the situation does not quite fit with our expectations. Yet it seems essential that we should ask about and listen to individual experiences and take into account people's perceptions as to what constitutes abuse and then act accordingly. As one American writer suggests, 'Abuse, like beauty is in the eye of the beholder' (Callahan, 1988, p. 454). There may be many different beholders (or witnesses) to abuse that happens in different care settings and we need to ensure that differing views and interpretations of abuse and mistreatment can be accommodated and dealt with appropriately. This also means that we must take into account the fact that the different witnesses may be quite likely to have different views about what would be an appropriate method of dealing with the situation. When researching abuse and individual experiences of abuse, however, it will be essential that clear and explicit definitions are made so that findings can be applied appropriately and consistently and limitations can be acknowledged.

ACTIVITY 2.2

Write a list of those people who might witness situations of abuse in a care home setting. Compare this to a list of those people who might witness abusive situations in a person's own home.

In your comparison of lists, you may have found some overlap, but there will also be some differences in terms of potential witnesses. Additionally the list for care home settings is likely to be longer than the one for the domestic (or home) setting as it probably includes members of care staff, other members of staff (such as those employed for catering or maintenance activities) and volunteers who visit the home.

The broadest definition of abuse that is in use in the UK at present is found in the Department of Health and Welsh Assembly Government documents, which were issued in 2000. This definition (shared in both documents) states:

> Abuse is the violation of an individual's human and civil rights by any other person or persons.
>
> (Department of Health, 2000a, para. 2.3)

On its own, however, this definition is not terribly helpful as it potentially includes a very wide range of actions. The guidance documents produced by government therefore also tried to make this somewhat clearer by following the definition with a discussion about the different types of abuse that can occur.

Types of abuse

Whilst it may remain difficult to define abuse, there is general agreement on the range of types and levels at which it is experienced. These include:

- physical abuse
- sexual abuse
- psychological abuse
- material abuse (which may include exploitation of finance or possessions)
- neglect (self-neglect or acts of omission of care).

Increasingly, this list is being extended to include acts that are institutionalised by the policies and practices of individual agencies. This may include poor professional care practice that has developed unilaterally without concern for individually sensitive responses to people's care needs (see Department of Health, 2000a). It may also include systemic level abuse, whereby the regime of the institution has developed in ways that are abusive to the residents. This demarcation of differing forms of institutional abuse and neglect is the approach taken by the Department of Health in its guidance on developing multi-agency policies and procedures for adult protection (Department of Health, 2000a). Box 2.1 outlines this classification of the different types of abuse.

BOX 2.1   CATEGORIES OF ABUSE

- **Physical abuse**, including hitting, slapping, pushing, kicking, misuse of medication, restraint or inappropriate sanctions;
- **Sexual abuse**, including rape and sexual assault or sexual acts to which the vulnerable adult has not consented, or could not consent or was pressurised into consenting;
- **Psychological abuse**, including emotional abuse, threats of harm or abandonment, deprivation of contact, humiliation, blaming, controlling, intimidation, coercion, harassment, verbal abuse, isolation or withdrawal from services or supportive networks;
- **Financial or material abuse**, including theft, fraud, exploitation, pressure in connection with wills, property or inheritance or financial transactions, or the misuse or misappropriation of property, possessions or benefits;

continued

- **Neglect and acts of omission**, including ignoring medical or physical care needs, failure to provide access to appropriate health, social care or educational services, the withholding of the necessities of life, such as medication, adequate nutrition and heating, and
- **Discriminatory abuse**, including racist, sexist or acts that are based on a person's disability or age, and other forms of harassment, slurs or similar treatment.

(Department of Health, 2000a)

This kind of classification offers an accessible way of considering acts that may be abusive without entering into a lengthy and irresolvable debate about the nature of abuse. The underlying premise for this list is the overall definition of abuse that is contained within the guidance. This states that abuse consists of acts which violate another person's human and civil rights. This is clearly a very broad definition potentially encompassing a wide range of many different situations. The guidance therefore develops this further by indicating that abuse may be something that is done to another person or to oneself or, indeed, may also be something that is omitted from being done by oneself or another person (see Box 2.2 below).

Additionally, there may be several people involved in the abusive acts. Although we commonly look at abuse as being acts between two individuals, the 'abuser' (or 'perpetrator') and the 'victim', it is possible that more than one 'abuser' is involved. This may perhaps especially be the case in the situation of abusive regimes that exist within institutional care and involve most if not all staff members. Equally in care settings, there may be more than one 'victim' of abuse. For example, in a situation of institutional or system level abuse in a care home setting it is possible that several, if not most, of the residents of the home will be affected by an abusive regime, although the impact of such abuse may vary between individuals.

ACTIVITY 2.3

Write a list of those people who might be involved in situations of abuse in a care home setting (as abusers or perpetrators). Compare this to a list of those people who might perpetrate abuse in a person's own home.

When you compared your different lists, you may have found some similarities in terms of potential abusers, but there will also be a number of differences in terms of the potential people involved in abusive acts and situations. As we saw in the previous activity, the list for care home settings is likely to be longer than the one for the domestic (or home) setting as it probably includes members of care staff, other residents of the home or other form of institution, volunteers who visit the home or other members of staff, such as those employed in non-care positions, in addition to family members and relatives, friends and neighbours who may (continue to) act abusively even although the setting is different.

It is important to acknowledge here that although we may have a sense that institutional settings are safe environments for vulnerable people to live in, this may be far from the case. So the idea that placement in a care home will serve to protect someone who has experienced abuse at home may not be accurate. We must also be aware that simply changing the setting in which the individual lives does not automatically mean that the person will not experience abuse or neglect in that different setting and in addition different forms of abuse or neglect might happen. So, for example, someone who has experienced physical and psychological abuse from members of their family at home may perhaps be quite well protected in a care home from continuing physical abuse by the family but the psychological abuse may continue if care is not taken in terms of visits and access. Alternatively, a different form of abuse, such as financial or material abuse or neglect may occur instead of the forms of abuse that occurred at home. What we are suggesting here is that care must be taken when considering institutional forms of care for people, perhaps especially for those who have experienced abuse in the domestic (or home) setting. This is important as early research by Eastman found that practitioners reported that when intervening they would favour finding an institutional placement for an older person who had been abused at home (Eastman, 1984). However, it is probably just as unwise to think that all institutions will act in ways that are abusive or neglectful as it is to consider that all institutions are safe places.

Whilst most UK categorisations of abuse, mistreatment and neglect do not often include matters of self-neglect, it is clear that leaving a vulnerable person in a known position or setting in which self-neglect is likely to happen may well constitute an act of omission, or indeed a service failure. It almost certainly leaves the individual in a vulnerable position or serves to increase their vulnerability and this is a factor to be taken into consideration when undertaking individual assessments.

BOX 2.2 DEFINITION OF ABUSE

Abuse may consist of a single act or repeated acts. It may be physical, verbal or psychological, it may be an act of neglect or an omission to act, or it may occur when a vulnerable person is persuaded to enter into a financial or sexual transaction to which he or she has not consented, or cannot consent. Abuse can occur in any relationship and may result in significant harm to or exploitation of, the person subjected to it.

(Department of Health, 2000a, para. 2.6)

Recognising discriminatory and racist abuse, as seen in the Department of Health list above in Box 2.1, is an important step forward. However, we can move wider still in seeking to understand abuse and also need to consider abuse that is structural and systemic (Pritchard, 2000). It is structural in that it is part of the fabric of society, in the myths and attitudes spread about vulnerable people and their particular vulnerabilities and characteristics and the discrimination that they may face in daily life. This may be particularly evident in the way that services are organised and provided and in the lack of value attached to groups who deviate from supposed norms of well-being and normality, as we will see in later chapters. Abuse can be considered to be systemic in being interactive and resulting from the actions of services with service users, carers and other groups. It can also be seen in the opportunities that this closes down for those in receipt of services and the meanings constructed by involvement within the care service systems. Where poor care or even neglect occurs frequently, it may indicate that the care setting itself is abusive. Indeed, 'repeated instances of poor care may be an indication of more serious problems and this is sometimes referred to as *institutional abuse*' (Department of Health, 2000a, para. 2.9).

It is important to note that the direction of abuse can be very important in the context of abuse in care settings. For instance, in an institutional setting abuse may occur from resident to resident, resident to staff, staff to resident and, introducing an aspect of social justice often forgotten, staff to staff (see Figure 2.1). This figure deals solely with institutional interpersonal abuse and excludes abuse from family members, relatives and acquaintances, volunteers or strangers, although we must acknowledge that within care settings abusive situations may also occur from the actions of others such as those listed above who act abusively or continue to act abusively within the care setting. And as indicated above, although care homes are often considered to be safe places for people to live in, especially if they have experienced abuse elsewhere, we know from scandals that have occurred that institutional (care) settings may also be very unsafe places for vulnerable adults who have a variety of care needs to live in and that abuse and abusive regimes may also occur in these places. Figure 2.1 also excludes possible abuse deriving from social care systems and practices, or from either policies or procedures guiding those services.

We also need to be aware that there are in fact many levels at which abuse can operate. These are illustrated in Figure 2.2. We must note here, however, that these levels interact and interconnect with one another.

These different dimensions at which abuse and abusive situations can operate may also be represented by reference to micro, mezzo and macro levels of abuse (see Bennett et al., 1997). Table 2.1 relates these different levels to types of abuse and possible causes within care settings. It is important for practitioners to develop the capacity to consider the interactions between these different levels in their daily practice. This helps both in explaining abuse and in deciding on the actions that need to be taken in order to counteract it.

There is a developing debate as to whether or not we should think of incidents of abuse in these areas in terms of their criminality rather than separating them into issues of welfare and the need for care services. *No Secrets* (Department of Health, 2000a) acknowledges that some abusive acts constitute criminal offences and indicates that when an allegation has been made any police criminal investigation must take precedence over other enquiries. This means it is imperative that practitioners in care settings have clear guidance and procedures to ensure that alleged criminal matters are referred to the police. The police may not always become directly involved in such situations; it may be sufficient at times just to consult with them, perhaps via a telephone conversation. In other circumstances, it may be that, after initial liaison and some quite brief involvement, the police do not continue to play a part in the ongoing processes. The important thing to remember here, in line with the guidance, is the need to consider whether police involvement may be needed as early as possible and to make sure that decisions are made in relation to this at an early stage in any assessment of an alleged abusive situation. This is in part to ensure that if a police investigation needs to take

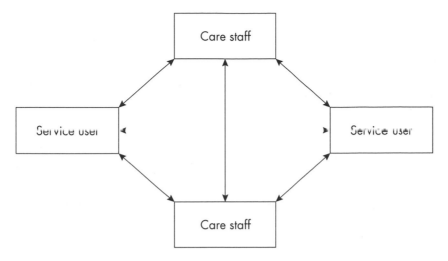

FIGURE 2.1 Directions of abuse in care settings

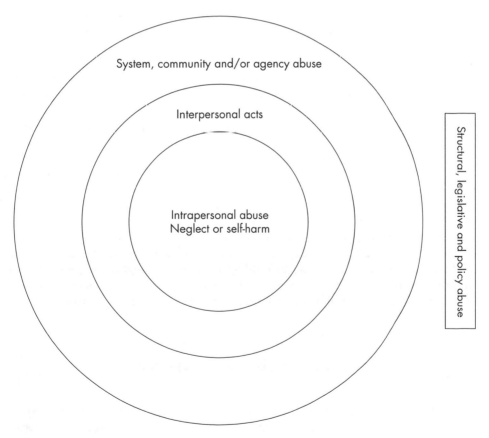

FIGURE 2.2 The levels of abuse

Table 2.1 The types and levels of abuse

Types of abuse	Macro level – political or structural	Mezzo level – community or agency	Micro level – individual
Abuse of vulnerable adults by professionals and care staff in care settings	Poor employment conditions Lack of effective selection and recruitment strategies or employment screening	Lack of training and education for care staff Poor management systems Poor levels of support and guidance	Work-related stress and professional burnout Psychopathology of individual staff members and/or service users Personal characteristics of 'victims'
Abuse in care settings (abusive regimes)	Societal expectations of a predominantly female and low-paid workforce Lack of social policy commitment to high-quality care Ambivalence of wider society regarding care for vulnerable adults	Lack of adequate resources to provide good-quality care Too few staff Isolation of institution from wider society	Staff work in isolation Inadequate guidance for care staff Low self-esteem of staff Personal characteristics of 'victims'

Source: adapted from Juklestad (2001) and Parker (2001).

place there will not be any difficulty arising from actions taken by someone else at an earlier point that could compromise the investigation (for instance, the failure to preserve evidence).

Brogden and Nijhar's (2000) arguments are important here. They suggest that the welfare argument of abuse, abuser and abused fails to lay responsibility for the acts with perpetrators and also marks out the victim of the crime as in some way 'needy'. Considering situations through a 'welfare lens' means that the orientation is predominantly about care, treatment and protection, rather than a perspective that focuses on justice or restitution. Furthermore, a failure to consider abuse or abusive situations as potential crimes may mean that the matter does not get dealt with in an appropriate way. If the criminal nature of what is currently termed 'abuse' was paramount, those committing such acts could be punished more readily under the law and the unacceptability of such acts would be confirmed throughout society. These are important arguments and ones which at the very least need to be incorporated into our understanding. The following case study illustrates some of the reasons.

CASE STUDY 2.2: HENRY

Henry Roberts was transferred to Blythe Way residential home when the local authority home he had been living in closed down. He had lived there for some three years, moving in after his wife had died. Henry did not communicate much, was described as still grieving for his wife but seemed to understand when spoken to. He had been known to masturbate openly in the visitors' room in the local authority home, which was dealt with by leading him away to his own room and making sure he knew this was unacceptable. This information was passed with him on his transfer to Blythe Way.

A few weeks after he had been placed at Blythe Way, the manager rang social services to demand that he should be either removed from the home or prescribed medication to reduce his libido. Henry had been found on four occasions inappropriately touching a woman resident. The social worker who was allocated the referral, Karen, worked with the home to find out whether Henry knew what he was doing, when he was doing it and to outline what was expected and permissible and what was not. On finding that Henry was aware that what he was doing was inappropriate, Karen suggested that the home set out clear expectations and provide him time and space to talk about his wife. She also asked the home to ensure that he knew if he were to touch the woman again it might constitute an assault and that they would have to inform the police to investigate if a crime had been committed. The home refused to agree to this plan saying that they would lose business if they did not deal with the situation immediately and therefore they would call the doctor and have medication prescribed for him in order to deal with the situation more rapidly. The home manager did not appear to realise that the solution that the home preferred might not really meet Henry's needs in this situation.

However, the abuse being considered here is associated with specific care settings and actions or inaction within those settings. It is therefore helpful to consider the range of acts, often criminal but sometimes interpersonally cruel or unprofessional, under the banner of abuse. We also need to be aware of some of the risk factors and possible causes of abuse in institutional care settings.

Risk factors in institutional care

A number of writers have considered potential risk factors in relation to care settings. Phillipson and Biggs (1995) provide a sound overview of these and develop ideas concerning risk factors. Those factors that have attracted most agreement include the following. The vulnerability of residents (care recipients) and their relative inability to protect themselves is seen as likely to increase the risk of abuse occurring. The existence of high levels of dependency, severe physical and/or cognitive limitations of residents, and potential communication difficulties, where individuals may not be able to express themselves or their feelings clearly, may also possibly intensify risk. Communication difficulties in the form of very poor systems of communication for staff may also worsen the problem. There are further factors relating to staff issues as we shall see below.

In addition, a lack of satisfactory systems for complaints may add to the risk of abuse not being detected or acted upon. Fear of retaliation, or of making the situation worse, may result in reluctance on the part of individuals to report or even talk about what is happening. This can include reticence on the part of relatives to intervene in a situation, or to raise issues concerning particular situations. Such aspects may be further compounded by both a lack of knowledge about the rights of residents and low expectations in relation to care standards from residents and their relatives. Many people may not know what to expect from care home settings and may also not be aware of what is acceptable behaviour or treatment or not. They may also believe, or in some instances even be told, that the staff are the experts and know best how to treat the people in their care. One of us (Penhale) remembers a situation early on in her social work career in the 1980s when social workers were told by senior social services management in a local authority that residential care staff knew best how to deal with challenging residents and difficult situations when questions were asked about why certain practices were used in a care home setting for disturbed adolescents. This home was subsequently (several years later) the subject of an abuse investigation concerning the treatment regimes used there.

Causes of abuse in institutional care

In his work looking at scandals and inquiries in institutional care settings in the UK, Clough has developed a number of ideas about the likely causes of abuse in those settings (Clough, 1996). Juklestad has also considered these and states:

> The causes of abuse are many and complex. It depends, to an extent on the type of abuse that is occurring; for example, whether it is an individual act or arising from an abusive regime in the institution.
>
> (Juklestad, 2001, p. 37)

However, it seems that the risk of abuse is likely to be greater in certain circumstances (see Box 2.3):

BOX 2.3   CAUSES OF ABUSE IN CARE SETTINGS

The staff:

- receive little support from the management
- lack training
- receive inadequate guidance
- have low self-esteem
- have poor personal standards
- work in isolation

The institution:

- has poor management
- has too few staff
- has little direction from the outside
- has poor communication with the world outside

(Juklestad, 2001, p. 38)

Clough has tended to concentrate on organisational issues as causative factors (Clough, 1996). The list that he has developed includes management failure and confused purposes or tasks as being of prime importance. Additionally, inadequate guidelines or training for staff in such areas as restraint use, risk taking and abuse are also highlighted as causing difficulties. The low status and morale of care staff are also a key area of concern: many staff working in care settings are very poorly paid, receive minimal training and may work in isolation or be part-time members of staff. The capacity of staff to work effectively with vulnerable adults, particularly if there are individuals who lack mental capacity, is also of concern. Staff members need to be trained in techniques relating to the provision of care and in how to give good standards of care. Yet in addition to being powerless to change many of the situations that they encounter, members of care staff may also be undervalued by the management.

Further factors that are involved include resource problems. Additionally, a lack of equipment resulting from such problems is likely to be linked to other difficulties relating to the appropriate treatment of service users. Furthermore, a failure on the part of regulators and inspectors to detect patterns or to monitor changes in care standards properly will add to problem areas. This could lead to the inability to detect and deal with difficulties at an early stage in their development. Attitudes and behaviour towards residents also play a part in this. If the organisational regime treats individuals as children and as if they are somehow not human, then care practices may become corrupt and abuse may result. One of us (Penhale) recalls visiting an old-style long-stay hospital for people with learning disabilities in the 1980s where the living conditions were very poor and there was a chronic lack of equipment. The hospital staff appeared unmotivated and even depressed by conditions. The hospital was in a rural setting and was quite isolated; many of the staff had accommodation located in the hospital grounds or very close by. Patients seemed to receive care at very basic levels (food, heat, etc.), but were generally not provided with activities or other forms of stimulation. A large number of the patients had lived at the hospital for many years and most staff did not think that the majority of them could be relocated to live in the community. Additionally, there seemed to be widespread attitudes that these adults could only live in a hospital environment and should be treated as if they were children. The hospital was later closed, partly because of an enquiry into standards of care due to complaints of physical abuse and neglect of patients' needs.

SUMMARY

In this chapter, we have considered the nature of vulnerability and also explored what constitutes abuse and neglect. We have included in this chapter a consideration of institutional abuse and abuse that happens in care settings as many social care workers will come into contact with institutions of one sort and another throughout their working lives. There has been a tendency to think of care settings as safe places, yet as we have seen it is possible that they may be quite dangerous places for vulnerable individuals to be in. Having considered the different types of abuse that may occur the next chapter moves to explore aspects of the law relating to adult protection.

KEY READING

Bennett, G., Kingston, P. and Penhale, B. (1997) *The Dimensions of Elder Abuse: Perspectives for Practitioners*, Basingstoke: Macmillan.

Clough, R. (1996) *Abuse of Care in Residential Institutions*, London: Whiting and Birch.

Department of Health (2000a) *No Secrets: Guidance on Developing and Implementing Multi-agency Policies and Procedures to Protect Vulnerable Adults from Abuse*, London: Department of Health.

Lord Chancellor's Department (1998) *Who Decides?: Making Decisions on Behalf of Mentally Incapacitated Adults*, London: The Stationery Office.

THE LAW

INTRODUCTION

Social work and social care practitioners operate within the boundaries of specific legislation, and the agencies in which they work often have a mandate derived from social welfare policies and legislation. This is the case for those working in voluntary and independent agencies as well as in the statutory sector. This chapter will discuss the ways in which practitioners can use law and policy in their practice in relation to adult protection.

It is often stated and bemoaned that there is no legislation comparable to the Children Act, 1989, that is specifically concerned with the protection of vulnerable adults. However, what is almost equally often neglected is the wide range of legislation that is available. The Economic and Social Research Council Violence

Research Programme overview (Stanko et al., 2002) lists fifty-nine separate statutes relevant to protection from violence and these have been added to since. These laws cover children as well as adults, relate to the four countries of the UK – England, Wales, Scotland and Northern Ireland – and are very wide-ranging. The fact that many of them do relate to adults, however, and are part of the general legislative framework for protecting people from abuse and harm, is important. There is perhaps within this situation a hint of the contest between a criminal justice approach in which acts are considered and treated as any other criminal act or assault and a welfare approach seeing acts as abuse which some may suggest minimises the magnitude of those acts (see Brogden and Nijhar, 2000). It is also the case, as we shall see later in this chapter, that moves are being made to ensure that adult protection is accorded greater emphasis, especially within the context of modernising social services and social and health care. Of course, questions may be asked as to why we have separate legislation relating to people solely on the basis of age but this raises a range of philosophical and social issues that are beyond the scope of the current debate. This chapter presents key aspects of contemporary legislation, policies and guidance that have been issued to assist practitioners in dealing with abuse and protection.

ACTIVITY 3.1

Spend a few moments listing those key pieces of legislation and social policy of which you are aware that could be used to protect adults who are vulnerable to or who have experienced abuse or harm. Use Table 3.1 to categorise this legislation. Keep this list whilst you work through the chapter and revise it as necessary. You may surprise yourself about your knowledge of legislation that can be used in adult protection!

Table 3.1 Legislation and safeguarding adults

	Social welfare legislation	*Criminal justice legislation*
Relates to adults only		
Relates to all people regardless of age		

The situation in Scotland is different to the other countries in the UK, with an Adult Support and Protection Bill being enacted in March 2007, which will provide powers to:

- set up new multi-agency adult protection committees to oversee local policies and their implementation
- place a duty on agencies to investigate abuse when it is suspected

- carry out an assessment of the person and their circumstances under certain conditions
- create a range of interventions to address and manage the abuse of vulnerable adults
- mandate health and social care agencies to work together.

The legislation that does exist in the UK may be conceptualised as a three-stage model of protection. It is aimed at preventing the risk of harm and abuse occurring, at targeting 'at risk' communities, groups and individuals and at dealing with abuse and harm after it has been committed. Of course, different parts of an Act may relate to different aspects of prevention or intervention and it is not always easy to identify clearly in which category the legislation stands.

ACTIVITY 3.2

Using your list of legislation that you have compiled in the previous activity, and thinking about the three categories – prevention, removal of risk, alleviation of further harm – see if you can highlight aspects of the legislation that fit into each category.

KEY ELEMENTS OF LEGISLATION TO PROTECT ADULTS FROM ABUSE

Key elements of legislation relevant in the protection of adults include the Offences Against the Person Act of 1861, which, although very old, allows for criminal acts of physical abuse and violence to be prosecuted. The Mental Health Act, 1983 (and proposed changes under the draft Mental Health Bill, 2006), provides protection for people with mental health problems who may be in danger of self-harm or, indeed, harming other people. The Protection from Harassment Act, 1997, relates to fear and harassment experienced by individuals because of the actions of others (Johns, 2005). These disparate Acts are useful and important in working to protect adults when abuse, harm or fear of harm is apparent. They are reactive to situations and events in which risk or harm has occurred, however, rather than developing a primary protective social system, one that seeks to prevent harm occurring by creating the conditions for social justice. It is the latter that we shall begin by considering.

Prevention and protection

In updating the National Assistance Act, 1948, the National Health Service and Community Care Act, 1990, details the duties of Councils with Social Service Responsibilities (CSSRs) to provide accommodation for people aged over eighteen years who need care and attention because of their age, illness or disability (S.42). However, the Act set out a wider protective function and provided for the development of community care services plans for the area (S.46). In compiling the plans, health services, housing services and voluntary organisations were to be consulted. There was a great optimism in this provision which, on the surface at least, addressed the needs of a community and the potential to provide services that would enable independence and choice, protecting people from situations which might make them vulnerable. However, the section made no allowance for the potential costs, the criteria for development and provision or standardised services to account for needs. This has plagued the Act since, and the development of a standardised framework to assist councils in setting eligibility criteria, under *Fair Access to Care Services* guidance (Department of Health, 2003a), may lead to the restriction of services in times of limited resources, reflecting more the creation of vulnerability than reducing it!

The personal aspects of the Act and the duty of the local authority are contained in section 47 which states the duty to carry out an assessment of needs and determine whether the needs require the provision of any services – but the judgement as to whether services should be provided is left with the local authority and subject, therefore, to economic and political constraint (see Mandelstam, 1999):

> S.47 (1) . . . where it appears to a local authority that any person for whom they may provide or arrange for the provision of community care services may be in need of any such services, the authority –
>
> (a) shall carry out an assessment of his needs for those services; and
> (b) having regard to the results of that assessment, shall then decide whether his needs call for the provision by them of any such services.

Modernisation and change in social and health care have underpinned the Labour government's vision since coming to power in 1997. They are seen as a means of improving services, eliminating waste and maximising the use of public funds (Department of Health, 1998a). The White Paper *Modernising Social Services* (Department of Health, 1998b) outlined the priorities for both adult and children's social services, placing emphasis on increased regulation as a means of better protecting service users and controlling workforce issues. This has continued throughout subsequent administrations. The White Paper *Our Health, Our Care, Our Say* (Department of Health, 2006a) takes the modernising and improvement agenda forward by shifting the focus toward fostering greater independence and well-being and having a choice about services but is clear that this will not be to the detriment of those needing protection:

> This [strategic shift] will not, however, be at the expense of those with high levels of need for whom high quality services – and, where necessary, protection for those unable to safeguard themselves – must be in place. In delivering this strategic shift, we are committed to a health and social care system that promotes fairness, inclusion and respect for people from all sections of society, regardless of their age, disability, gender, sexual orientation, race, culture or religion, and in which discrimination will not be tolerated.
>
> (Department of Health, 2006a, p. 17, para. 1.27)

Preventative, or primary, approaches to protection are seen throughout the White Paper and it is important for social care workers to be involved in promoting and working with such measures. Health promotion and the quality of the environment are central to well-being, and environmental planning and design are fundamental here. The overall vision for social care in the White Paper is laudable:

> B.4 Over the next 10 to 15 years, we want to work with people who use social care to help them transform their lives by:
>
> - Ensuring they have more control;
> - Giving them more choices and helping them decide how their needs can be met;
> - Giving them a chance to do the things that other people take for granted;
> - Giving them the best quality of support and protection to those with the highest levels of need.
>
> (Department of Health, 2006a, p. 204)

As well as this overall approach, the White Paper recognises the need to address at-risk groups in respect of violence and workplace stress (para. 2.40), in respect of domestic violence by identifying abuse and encouraging multidisciplinary responses to it (para. 4.79–80).

ACTIVITY 3.3

In what ways might you as a social care practitioner be part of a drive to improve social justice? Do you think that individual social care workers should be involved in such political activities and, if so, how might they go about this in their professional roles?

Protection from others

The Family Law Act, 1996, is also relevant when working with vulnerable adults, especially those experiencing domestic violence. This Act provides greater recognition of the rights and needs of people at risk from partners and relatives. It needs to be recognised that older people, people with physical health problems, mental illness, learning disabilities and so forth may be affected by and may perpetrate domestic violence. The Domestic Violence, Crime and Victims Act, 2004, represents an important addition to legislation available to protect people and prevent further abuse. The Act makes common assault (any intentional or reckless action that uses unlawful force or violence, Criminal Justice Act, 1988, S.39) an arrestable offence, and provides the police powers to arrest, as a criminal offence, a breach of a non-molestation order punishable by up to five years in prison. It also extends the protection gained from non-molestation and occupation orders under the Family Law Act, 2005, to same-sex couples and extends the availability of orders to people who have not cohabited or married.

There is, under section 5 of the Act, a new offence of familial homicide, of 'causing or allowing the death of a child or vulnerable adult', which came into force in March 2005. The intention was to close a legal loophole to prevent jointly accused people of escaping justice by remaining silent or blaming each other for the situation. The new offence allows the person causing the death and the person who knew this was happening but did not prevent it to bear some criminal responsibility. For the person who witnessed but did not prevent the crime, their situation is as an accessory to the crime. The offence is considered so serious as to carry up to fourteen years' imprisonment. There are some concerns about this law further abusing or failing to protect already frightened and vulnerable people. If a person can show they took reasonable steps to protect the person who died, and if that person was subject to domestic violence, this may be a factor in mitigation, but the expectation is clear that people must take reasonable steps to protect others who are vulnerable and at risk. It is hoped that it will also mean that the death of a vulnerable adult in the domestic setting may be more likely to result in a prosecution.

CASE STUDY 3.1: MARGARET

Margaret Bowlby lived with her son, James, and second husband, Stan. As Stan became increasingly frail and his physical health needs grew, James began to limit or deny his medication. Margaret was aware of this but did not intervene or tell anyone about this. James had told her she would 'get what for' if she mentioned it. Stan died as a result of heart failure exacerbated by not taking his medication.

Do you think the 2004 Act is relevant to this case study?

The Sexual Offences Act, 2003, is particularly important in respect of the protection of adults with a 'mental disorder' which renders such a person unable to refuse to take part in or witness a sexual act because they lack the capacity to agree or are unable to communicate their choices (S.30). Offences that involve penetration are taken extremely seriously under the Act and, on conviction, are punishable by life imprisonment.

It is an offence to incite or cause a person who cannot choose to engage in sexual activity as much as to engage directly in that activity with the person (S.31), or indeed to engage in sexual activity in the presence of people with a 'mental disorder' (S.32) or to cause them to watch sexual activity (S.33). Inducement, threat or deception to procure sexual activity is also noted as an offence (SS.34–7) in the same ways.

This Act is interesting and important for social care workers as it refers directly to care workers, fairly broadly defined, and sexual offences with a person with a 'mental disorder'. The subsection to the offences states:

> Where in proceedings for an offence under this section it is proved that the other person had a mental disorder, it is to be taken that the defendant knew or could reasonably have been expected to know that person had a mental

disorder unless sufficient evidence is adduced to raise an issue as to whether he knew or could reasonably have been expected to know it.

(SS.38–41 subsection 2)

Thus the Act seeks to protect vulnerable people from an abuse of power, and specifically adds protection from abuse by those with care responsibilities.

Protecting self and others

The Mental Health Act, 1983

It is important to mention the Mental Health Act in a little more depth. At present, social workers play a central role under the Mental Health Act, 1983, to protect people from harm to self or others arising from mental health difficulties. In this sense the Act serves a preventive function. Approved Social Workers (ASWs) – (to be known as Approved Mental Health Practitioners AMHPs under the proposed Bill) – act as independent assessors where it is thought that someone ought to be detained in hospital because of his or her mental health status. Whilst there is an increasing emphasis on working together more effectively with other professionals, especially given the development of integrated mental health services, there are strong arguments for retaining the independence of approved social workers. This serves to protect the rights of people with mental health problems who are at risk of being detained in hospital and thus, again, prevent potential 'abuse' from arising from structural or systemic misconceptions of mental illness. ASWs are also able, of course, to assist with the smooth admission to hospital for those who need hospital assessment or treatment and in ensuring that relatives and carers are supported and have the relevant information to challenge decisions made.

For some time, the Mental Health Act, 1983, has been under review; this process was originally begun in July 1998. A White Paper was published in 2000 (Department of Health, 2000b) which set out the government's intentions to reform mental health legislation, and a draft Mental Health Bill was published in 2002. This led to further consultation and a further revised draft Bill was published both in 2004 and in 2006. Some dangers within the proposed reforms are articulated well by the response of the Mental Health Special Interest Group of BASW (www.basw.co.uk/mhsig). The Bill proposes to replace the ASW with an Approved Mental Health Professional, who need not be a social worker and could, indeed, work for the Trust recommending in-patient assessment or treatment. This potential conflict of interests has not undergone significant debate (CSIP, 2005). The dangers of losing an independent role are clear. It could leave wide open the possibility that people could be compulsorily admitted to hospital without any recourse to independent assessment and thus have their liberty denied without the involvement of an independent person. The dilemma can be illustrated by the following case example.

CASE STUDY 3.2: OLDHAM WARD

Oldham Ward, a semi-secure psychiatric ward, called to arrange an Approved Social Work assessment of a man described as being actively suicidal, hallucinating and in need of being kept on the ward. He had been transferred from prison in the last few days of his sentence after trying to electrocute himself by inserting his fingers in the light bulb socket and standing in water. He had not realised that the voltage in cells had been lowered.

The ASW spoke with the man, who appeared rational, articulate and clear in his reasons for his actions. He said that he had been mistaken for a paedophile – his offences were in fact driving-related – and other inmates had begun threatening him. He said that he had become so frightened that he thought it better to kill himself rather than allow the other prisoners to get to him. The ASW checked the details of the story, spoke to ward staff, to his partner at home and formed the opinion that there was no reason for compulsorily detaining him in hospital. The ASW had a long discussion with the psychiatrist about this matter, finally getting him to agree in principle that there were no grounds to keep the man in hospital.

It is perhaps less likely that someone employed within the same organisation, working within the same managerial structures would be able to argue for this man's rights as effectively as an independent ASW.

The revised draft Bill, therefore, has improved potential safeguards that might be lost by requiring independent tribunal or court authorisation of compulsory detention after twenty-eight days. However, debates continue about the capacity issues required to service the number of tribunals that would be needed.

Also, we must note that structural issues of racism permeate the operation of the Act, with Black African and Caribbean people being three times more likely to be admitted as psychiatric in-patients and 44 per cent more likely to be compulsorily detained, suggesting a need to protect black and minority ethnic groups from abuse by the very legislation that has been developed to protect vulnerable people (www. healthcarecommission.gov.uk, Golightley, 2006).

The Mental Capacity Act, 2005

This Act gained its Royal Assent on 7 April 2005 after a long process of research and consultation. The intentions of the Act are to provide a statutory framework to protect vulnerable people who are not able to make decisions for themselves. The Act clarifies who can take decisions for and on behalf of these people, under what circumstances and how the process should take place, whilst allowing for some forward planning prior to the person's losing capacity. Because the Act is potentially powerful, those who have a professional duty to act under it, including social workers, will have to have work to guidance provided in the Code of Practice (Department for Constitutional Affairs, 2007, S.40 [4–5]).

The principles underlying the Act are important for social workers and social care practitioners as they state the 'presumption of capacity' unless proved otherwise and demand the provision of appropriate support to make decisions even when seen as eccentric or unwise. Where people no longer have the capacity to make decisions, anything that is done must be in their best interests and should be the least restrictive option in respect of their rights and freedoms. These principles have resonance with the value base of social work (Beckett and Maynard, 2005).

When assessing capacity, it is important to note that medical condition or diagnosis is not a sufficient test, nor is age, appearance or behaviour; the intention of this is to protect vulnerable people from unjustified assumptions and acts. But the Act also protects social workers and other professionals in stating that care can be provided for people who lack capacity, ensuring that medication can be provided and necessary goods, food and suchlike can be bought with their money. Where necessary to prevent harm to the person, restraint and restriction of liberty can be used proportionate 'to the likelihood and seriousness of the harm' (S.6). Restraint use must however be in line with existing guidance that exists about this.

The Act also creates 'lasting powers of attorney' (LPAs) to appoint someone to take decisions on behalf of a person if they lose capacity in the future, allowing the appointed person to make health and welfare decisions. Under the previous system of Powers and Enduring Powers of Attorney, decisions about health and welfare matters were not included. Under the new arrangements, the Public Guardian will co-ordinate and register LPAs and work with the Court of Protection as the final arbiter of the Act. There are further provisions in the Act to protect vulnerable people. An Independent Mental Capacity Advocate (IMCA) can be appointed for people lacking capacity but having no one to speak for them and requiring an advocate. This will include individuals who lack capacity but may need assistance in relation to adult protection processes. In fact this service will be available to individuals even if they have family or relatives who might be able to assist but who would benefit from independent advice and assistance concerning adult protection matters. It will also be available for either a victim of abuse or the abuser (or both) where these individuals lack capacity. A new criminal offence of ill-treatment or neglect of a person who lacks capacity was introduced by the Act, from April 2007, carrying a prison term of up to five years.

According to the Code of Practice, professionals acting under the Act must interact with relevant agencies for the protection of vulnerable adults either at risk of or experiencing abuse. The definition of abuse used in the Code of Practice is taken from the *No Secrets* and *In Safe Hands* guidance demonstrating a 'joined-up' approach.

The Care Standards Act, 2000

Current social care legislation reflects the government's modernising agenda, which set out proposed developments in services. One of these concerned improvements in the protection of people, both adults and children. The emphasis on protection in the *Modernising Social Services* White Paper (Department of Health, 1998b) is continued in Part VII of the Care Standards Act, 2000, which relates specifically to protection. This section of the Act covers issues of protection of both children and adults, but by far the majority of Part VII concerns the protection of vulnerable adults. It is of particular relevance to abuse that occurs in social care settings.

The Act defines 'care workers' in section 80 (2), stating a care worker to be 'an individual who is or has been employed in a position' enabling regular contact with adults who are accommodated in residential care, receiving hospital or clinic services (independent or National Health Service), or receiving personal care in their homes. Whilst day centres and voluntary clubs and groups are not specifically described, it is clear that, in relation to protection for vulnerable adults, the scope is meant to encompass all possible care settings.

A central aspect of the Care Standards Act is to make provision for a list of people considered to be 'unsuitable to work with vulnerable adults' (S.81 [1]) to be kept by the Secretary of State. This is known as the Protection of Vulnerable Adults (POVA) List and is similar to the list in operation for individuals who work with children, which was established under the Protection of Children Act, 1999. There were some delays in setting up the list for adults and operational difficulties are recognised; the list was introduced in July 2004. Stephen Ladyman's foreword to the guidance about the POVA List sets out the rationale and aims of the scheme:

> The Protection of Vulnerable Adults scheme will act as a workforce ban on those professionals who have harmed vulnerable adults in their care. It will add an extra layer of protection to the pre-employment processes . . . It will complement the Government's drive to raise standards across health and social care. Raising standards is an end in itself, but it is also the best way to protect vulnerable adults who, when they are harmed, are usually harmed because of care professionals' lack of knowledge or skill rather than out of malice.
>
> (Department of Health, 2004, p. 3)

However, the criteria set out in the guidance for referral for inclusion on the list included the following:

- dismissal for misconduct that harmed or placed at risk of harm a vulnerable adult; or for a worker who retires, resigns or is made redundant in similar circumstances who would have been otherwise dismissed
- transfer of the worker for the above reasons to a job not involving care
- suspension or temporary removal from care responsibilities whilst making a decision.

The intention here was that it would also be possible to make a referral when information comes to light in the future. Information is be gathered by the Secretary of State from the worker and the care provider in deciding whether to confirm inclusion of the individual's name on the list. The grounds to be satisfied concern a reasonable consideration of guilt of misconduct or that the worker is deemed unsuitable to work with vulnerable adults because they have harmed, or put at risk of harm, a vulnerable adult (or adults). The list is not retrospective, so that individuals with a previous dismissal or disciplinary action in relation to the harm of a vulnerable adult or adults could not be included on the list when it was set up. Referrals to the list could therefore be made only from the point of implementation of section 82 (26 July 2004) not before.

Employers, care worker provider agencies and registration authorities are empowered by the legislation to make referrals when certain conditions are met.

Procedures for dealing with staff who are the focus of an allegation of abuse are referred to in *No Secrets* (Department of Health, 2000a). Once a person has been referred for inclusion on the list, an inquiry is undertaken to determine whether there is sufficient evidence of misconduct or unsuitability to work with vulnerable adults (SS.83–5). This inquiry includes representation from the individual themselves about the situation and the opportunity to provide evidence in mitigation and to explain the circumstances surrounding the situation. If certain initial criteria are met the person's name is provisionally listed as a temporary measure whilst further inquiries and a decision about permanent listing take place.

As the legislation stands, individuals who are included on the list do have the right of appeal against inclusion. They can also make an application for removal from the list after five years if they were a child at the time of inclusion or ten years if they were an adult at the time that their name was added to the list.

The effects of inclusion on the list also mean that employers have to check people against the list prior to confirming an offer of employment. If an employer discovers later that an employee is on the list, the employer must cease to employ them. It is an offence for anyone on the list to work in a care position. The penalties for doing so will be a fine, imprisonment or both unless the person can prove they did not or could not know they were included on the list. However, as seen above, as part of the process of inclusion of names on the list, individuals are contacted by the Secretary of State and given the opportunity to comment on the statements or allegations made. In this way, it ought not to be possible for someone to say that they could not have known that their name was included on the list.

The Protection of Children Act, 1999, has been amended by the Care Standards Act to ensure compatibility with the protection of vulnerable adults. Individuals included on the POCA list as being unsuitable to work with children are also considered as to whether they are also unsuitable for working with vulnerable adults and vice versa. The Act also allows for cross-referrals if the misconduct appears to make a person unsuitable. As we will see below, this will be replaced by a unified system covering both children and adults, under the Safeguarding Vulnerable Groups Act, 2006.

The White Paper *Our Health, Our Care, Our Say* (Department of Health, 2006a) heralds the work of the Department for Education and Skills and the Department of Health to introduce the necessary legislation to create a new and streamlined vetting and barring system to prevent people from access to vulnerable people by taking paid or unpaid employment. The new scheme will build on the existing checks available through POVA and responds to the concerns of the Bichard Inquiry (2004). This inquiry was set up following the deaths of schoolgirls Holly Wells and Jessica Chapman in Cambridgeshire in 2002 and the subsequent convictions of Ian Huntley and Maxine Carr. The inquiry established that Huntley, who had been working as a school caretaker at the school that the girls attended, had not been adequately police-checked prior to commencing his post and also that 'soft police information' (relating to concerns rather than convictions) had not been passed from one police authority to another, or even retained on records relating to Huntley.

Safeguarding Vulnerable Groups Act, 2006

Recommendation 19 of the Bichard Inquiry concerning vetting and barring resulted in the introduction of the Safeguarding Vulnerable Groups Bill, which passed through Parliament in 2006 and received Royal Assent in late 2006. It will come into effect from 2008. The clearly stated aim of the vetting and barring scheme is to reduce the incidence of harm to children and vulnerable adults by helping to ensure that:

- employers benefit from an improved vetting service for those who work with children and/or vulnerable adults
- those people who are known to be unsuitable are barred from working with children and/or vulnerable adults at the earliest possible time.

The model that was proposed by government in response to the Bichard recommendation was subject to consultation during the summer of 2005. By far the majority of the respondents to the consultation (some 88 per cent) agreed with the suggested proposals and thought that the new scheme as proposed would have a positive effect on improving safeguards for children and vulnerable adults (Department of Health, 2006a).

The aims of the new scheme are to:

- build on the existing lists of those barred from work with children and vulnerable adults, including the POVA list
- be more comprehensive in coverage, with a wider workforce eligible for checks (including volunteers in some situations)
- enable a barring decision to be made on the basis of an individual's criminal record history, as well as following a referral from an employer or another body
- update barring decisions as soon as any new information is made available and notify employers if an employee is subsequently deemed unsuitable
- enable employers to make instant, secure, online checks of person's status in relation to the scheme.

Under the current proposals, individuals who commit certain listed offences will be automatically barred from working with children (and also in some cases vulnerable adults) with no right of appeal about this. For certain other offences, there is an automatic bar imposed, which an individual can appeal against in terms of their inclusion on the list of barred individuals. For further, more minor offences and situations an individual can be referred for consideration for inclusion on the list. The Act was passed during the 2006–7 parliamentary session and it is proposed that it will be implemented from 2008.

The provisions of the Care Standards Act, and specifically the provisions relating to the Protection of Vulnerable Adults, are to be welcomed. However, it must be noted that they are reactive measures that seek to remove or prevent unsuitable people from being in care positions. Of course, this will not necessarily prevent abuse from happening in care settings and therefore other measures will remain needed. Some of the frameworks, standards and guidance which have been developed go some way towards meeting this need.

ACTIVITY 3.4

Take a few moments to think about the vetting and barring scheme. If you were involved in drawing up a list of offences where there was an automatic bar to working with either children or vulnerable adults, with NO right of appeal against this, which offences would you include on the list? You may also wish to look at the information about the new scheme that appears on the Department of Health website (http://www.dh.gov.uk).

Towards ethical practice

What is important here is the recognition that effective intervention in working to protect vulnerable people is not simply the responsibility of individual practitioners. It is essential that all agencies involved in social and health care play an active role and that agencies are committed to working together in a systematic way to protect vulnerable individuals. It is also fundamental to good practice that structural changes occur, which shift public attitudes and social policies towards acknowledging the citizenship rights of vulnerable people. Whilst it may be beyond the scope of individual practitioners in social care settings to change society, it is a maxim of good practice that practitioners work towards social justice for individuals, within agencies and also in broader political terms. How can this be achieved? The collection of service user views, the inclusion of service user and carer perspectives in setting up and delivering services can be aided and promoted by practitioners. Support can be offered to help service users and carers speak up for themselves.

Also, the Public Interest Disclosure Act, 1998, and the Care Standards Act, 2000, demand that social care practitioners should report misgivings and concerns about practice in a way that can challenge existing practices. The often very real fears that practitioners in busy care settings have of speaking out about bad practice cannot be minimised. However, it is this concern weighed against the values and codes of practice outlined by the GSCC and by professional organisations such as BASW that must be considered. Work in care settings is seldom easy, but effective and ethical care demands that we take a stand when poor practice is identified. It is, however, also important that professional bodies and agencies respond to the challenges raised by the strength of an alliance of service users, carers and social care practitioners working towards social justice for all. National Minimum Standards for care agencies and settings have been published in recent years, to which social care practitioners and agencies are bound to subscribe. The authority for this is contained in section 23 of the Care Standards Act, 2000, as follows:

(1) The appropriate Minister may prepare and publish statements of national minimum standards applicable to establishments or agencies.
(2) The appropriate Minister shall keep the standards set out in the statements under review and may publish amended statements whenever he considers it appropriate to do so.
(3) Before issuing a statement, or an amended statement which in the

opinion of the appropriate Minister effects a substantial change in the standards, the appropriate Minister shall consult any persons he considers appropriate.

(4) The standards shall be taken into account –

    (a) in the making of any decision by the registration authority under this Part;

    (b) in any proceedings for the making of an order under section 20;

    (c) in any proceedings on an appeal against such a decision or order; and

    (d) in any proceedings for an offence under regulations under this Part.

In an attempt to follow through the rationale of developing National Minimum Standards that relate to different elements of social care, such as domiciliary and residential provision, in 2005 the Association for Directors of Social Services (ADSS) produced a document relating to Adult Protection. The document discussed a national framework for standards on Adult Protection (ADSS, 2005). This included a change in terminology, to Safeguarding Adults, following the trend established in relation to children and young people who experience abuse. This guidance from ADSS produced some interesting ideas concerning partnership working, responding to abuse and neglect and also preventing abusive and/or neglectful situations from arising, but has not been adopted as national level guidance, or fully endorsed by the Department of Health, so remains as optional for local authorities as to whether they choose to follow the guidance or not. The change in terms has also not been wholly adopted throughout the country.

Registered Homes Act, 1984

Before concluding this chapter about legislation and policy matters, we must also briefly discuss the Registered Homes Act, 1984. This Act is a key piece of legislation concerning residential and nursing home care provision and was introduced in order to introduce a regulatory framework for these care settings and to ensure appropriate standards of care. Private residential and care homes with nursing are licensed to operate under the Registered Homes Act, 1984, and action concerning registration is taken within the Act. Registration can be refused on three different grounds:

- 'Fit person': including the attitudes and values of individual owners and/or managers
- 'Fit premises': including physical accommodation; staffing ratios; equipment; state of repair
- Underlying philosophy: aims and objectives of the establishment and how care is provided within this.

Under the terms of the legislation, all registered homes with three or more residents must be inspected on an annual basis. The inspection and registration of small homes (with fewer than three residents) is covered within separate legislation, which was introduced later. Guidance states that ideally, there should be two visits by inspectors to registered care homes each year, at least one of which should be unannounced. Nursing and residential homes inspectors are now employed by the Commission for

Social Care Inspection (CSCI) and their remit also covers care provision from the statutory sector (for example, NHS nursing homes and social services residential care provision). There was some discussion and debate during 2005–6 concerning a proposal by government to reduce the inspection system to a system of 'proportionality' so that the frequency of inspections is based on the assessment and evaluation of how well an establishment is achieving the standards of care that have been set. In addition there is a suggestion that all inspection visits should be unannounced in order to check effectively on the performance of establishments.

As part of the current existing arrangements of the annual inspection process, there should be a review of the registration criteria (i.e. are all three elements still complied with?). Failure under any of the criteria can be used in the determination of cancellation of registration. There are two main ways that this is achieved: either through an emergency closure order (which uses section 11 of the Act and is used only in extreme circumstances), or a longer-term route to cancellation (using section 10 of the Act). These will be outlined briefly below.

Under section 10 of the Registered Homes Act, 1984, an application for registration of a home may be refused or registration cancelled if a person or premises are considered 'unfit', or if the underlying philosophy is no longer appropriate. If an inspection by the inspectors highlights a problem, then attempts should be made by the inspector to work with the owner to rectify the situation (unless an emergency closure is warranted under section 11; see below). This will require the owner to be given legal notice of the problem, through a Regulation 20 notice in a letter, and what steps should be taken to resolve it within a given time period.

If the home owner persistently fails to comply with regulations or to resolve identified problems within a set time, their registration licence may be revoked. Alternatively, an owner may be prosecuted in a Magistrate's court concerning a specific problem, which does not necessarily result in cancellation of the registration. If cancellation of the registration is decided on by the court, there are rights of appeal by the owner against cancellation to local councillors and to Registered Homes Tribunals who can uphold either the appeal or the cancellation of registration.

A number of criticisms of the 1984 Registered Homes Act have been made (Brammer, 1999). Within the Act itself, the term 'unfit' is not defined. Some remedies to problems have been suggested (Brammer, 1999). For example, with regard to the 'fit person criteria', Brammer suggests that a statutory definition of 'unfitness', alongside a checklist of factors to be considered in establishing 'fitness', would help with decision-making processes (Brammer, 2006).

In situations where there is a 'serious risk to the life, health, or well being of residents in a home', a magistrate may make an order cancelling registration with immediate effect (under section 11 of the Registered Homes Act). The registration authority (now the CSCI) usually makes application to the magistrate. This application can be made *ex parte*, without the owner knowing about the intended action beforehand.

This type of emergency action does however mean that the home can no longer operate. The effect is immediate closure and the residents have to move to other accommodation, with all the trauma that this involves for the residents, who are usually already vulnerable. Whilst this somewhat drastic action may be in the best interests of the residents in the long term, it is sometimes difficult for inspectors who are aware of the difficulties of transferring perhaps more than a hundred residents to alternative accommodation. The inspectors may therefore require very high levels of proof prior to taking action regarding closure. In some situations, although the home owners and management may be prevented from continuing to run the home, an alternative management system, perhaps provided by the local CSSR, may be put in place in the home until more permanent arrangements can be made.

It is also necessary to acknowledge that inspection units must work closely with other agencies when there are allegations of abuse within homes. An inspector will generally only conduct an investigation concerning a possible breach of registration criteria (although this may concern an abusive regime within the home). A parallel police investigation may be necessary, for example, concerning an assault of an individual resident. In addition, in many areas, it is likely that any reports of alleged abuse of an individual will be passed to a district social work or care management team to deal with. This is because the registration authority is mainly concerned with those aspects which directly concern them (for instance in determining whether a breach of registration criteria occurred). It is hoped, however, the further development of the CSCI and its successor organisation when the CSCI joins with the Commission for Healthcare Improvement (CHAI) and the Mental Health Act Commission (MHAC) in 2008, and the existing government emphasis on improving protection for vulnerable people, will result in changes to this situation.

Ethical practice, which serves to protect vulnerable service users, is as essential for health and social care practitioners and within care settings as elsewhere. The emphasis found within *No Secrets* on system level and institutional abuse represents a welcome recognition, at the level of government, that abuse in care settings is an issue of key importance when considering adult protection (Department of Health, 2000a). For practitioners, knowledge of the appropriate legislative and policy documents is therefore very necessary and fundamental as a prerequisite to good practice.

SUMMARY

In this chapter we have reviewed the key aspects of legislation and social policy that influence approaches to working with abuse in care settings and that can be used to assist people who have been abused or to prevent others from abusing. Whilst there is no single piece of legislation, it is clear that there are many different Acts, now supplemented by a concerted policy effort aimed at increasing protection, that social care practitioners can use. However, not everyone will have access to such diverse knowledge or to a legal team who can assist. There is a need for training on an ongoing and regular basis and, indeed, a professional responsibility to update knowledge. It is the use of such practice-oriented policy documents as *No Secrets* (Department of Health, 2000a) that can best assist here. Co-ordination between agencies and clarity in decision-making across and within agencies has the potential to help guide practice to protect people in vulnerable situations.

KEY READING

ADSS (2005) *Safeguarding Adults: A National Framework of Standards for Good Practice and Outcomes in Adult Protection Work*, London: Association of Directors of Social Services.

Brammer, A. (2006) *Social Work Law* (2nd edition), Harlow: Pearson.

Brayne, H. and Carr, H. (2005) *Law for Social Workers* (9th edition), Oxford: Oxford University Press.

Johns, R. (2007) *Using the Law in Social Work* (3rd edition), Exeter: Learning Matters.

Johns, R. and Sedgwick, A. (1998) *Law for Social Work Practice: Work with Vulnerable Adults*, Basingstoke: Macmillan.

Smith, K. and Tilney, S. (2007) *Vulnerable Adult and Child Witnesses*, Oxford: Blackstone.

CHAPTER 4

PERFORMANCE MANAGEMENT, INSPECTION, REGULATION AND QUALITY ASSURANCE ISSUES

OBJECTIVES

By the end of the chapter you should:

- understand the place of quality assurance, inspection, regulation and performance management in contemporary social work and social care

- be able to describe key elements of the regulatory process

- be able to think how the processes of monitoring may assist in the protection of adults

- be able to identify and critique some of the potential drawbacks of performance management, regulation and inspection for person-centred care and adult protection

- be able to consider ways of assuring the quality of and enhancing one's own practice.

INTRODUCTION

The world of social and health care has developed a complex set of structures aimed at ensuring that service provision meets core standards, and that care is improved to meet needs. These worthy aims are set within a context of finite resources and the requirement to provide cost-effective and efficient services. There are tensions here, of course, which are clearly played out within and between three levels of social care: the macro level at which performance measures, targets and overall budgets pre-dominate; the agency, team or mezzo level in which local need confronts given budgets;

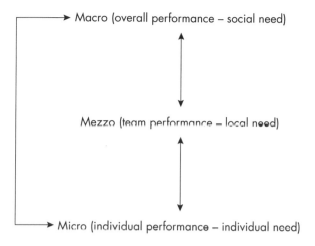

FIGURE 4.1 The interactions between the three levels of service performance and monitoring

the individual professional or micro level in which service user's and carer's needs are balanced against the remit of the team, competing claims for resources across those requiring a service, and professional values (see Figure 4.1).

The permeation of monitoring technologies and the concomitant rise in the visibility of social care practices have characterised organisational developments and changes in legislation over the last few decades. As a means of improving quality this emphasis becomes clear when, in 1984, the Registered Homes Act provided for the scrutiny and registration of care homes (see Chapter 3). The intention behind this legislation lay in a wish to ensure that care in homes for vulnerable people and the personal care provided safeguarded and promoted the welfare of residents (Mandelstam, 1999).

The emphasis on accountability, registration and increased 'visibility' of care practices grew rapidly in the last two decades of the twentieth century. The National Health Service and Community Care Act, 1990, and subsequent guidance underscored the importance of monitoring and inspection and the assurance of quality in social and health care as a preferred means of enhancing practice by the regulation of standards. The prominence given to these aspects of provision was continued and given fresh impetus by the 1997 Labour government's modernising agenda that has emphasised service improvement through monitoring and regulation (Department of Health, 1998b). The Care Standards Act, 2000, crystallised the importance of this culture of visibility and accountability which was enshrined in the establishment of such inspection and monitoring bodies as the Commission for Social Care Inspection (CSCI) and regulatory bodies like the General Social Care Council (GSCC) (see Figure 4.2). The intention to protect vulnerable adults through the scrutiny of social care services and via the regulation of the workforce and social work education is a mainstay of government policy though the evidence base has not been subject to test. The continued belief in the efficacy of inspection and monitoring processes is clearly articulated within the adult health and social care White Paper, *Our Health, Our Care, Our Say* (Department of Health, 2006a). The evaluation of service provision and including the perspectives of service users as 'experts by experience' has become centrally important to both the

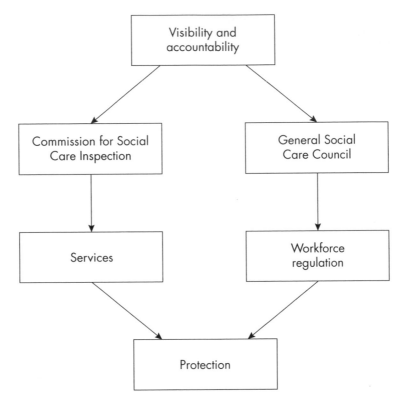

FIGURE 4.2 The culture of visibility and accountability in care services

commissioners and providers of services and forms part of the drive to ensure that suitable and effective measures are in place to regulate the provision of social care.

In this chapter we set the scene by providing an overview of key elements of inspection, monitoring and quality assurance, consider this in the context of performance management in which social workers and social care practitioners operate, explore the likely impact on working practices in teams and agencies and describe the importance of quality assurance and enhancement of individual practice. Evidence-based practice and practitioner research or evaluation are discussed as contributing to our approaches to matters of protection in social care with vulnerable adults.

SOCIAL WORK AND THE LOCAL AUTHORITIES

The regulation of social services and social work is bi-directional. Webb (2006) explains that, whilst social work as an activity is increasingly regulated, it too acts as a regulator of social life. We saw this when discussing the place of legislation in adult protection (see Chapter 3).

ACTIVITY 4.1

Think of some of the ways in which social work and social welfare are regulated and identify ways in which social work and welfare regulates social life. Write down some of these in two columns and compare the similarities and differences in each column. The following case study illustrates some of these issues.

CASE STUDY 4.1:   IMRAN

Imran, a social worker in a sensory impairment team, was due for his annual appraisal. His line manager advised him that he should undertake a post-qualifying award in social work and suggested that this would be helpful to him as he could gain a postgraduate degree over time. Imran reminded him that he already had a master's degree in social work and asked for training instead that would help him decide when to provide services even when they were not wanted or requested! In the debate his line manager acknowledged that the agency was trying to ensure a certain proportion of staff holding post-qualifying awards and Imran acknowledged he wanted an easy-step guide to negotiate the tensions of daily practice.

The principles of the modernising agenda in social and health care focus on service improvements, raising quality and responsiveness and ensuring that people who are made vulnerable by society or who for a variety of reasons are in need of protection are afforded the best possible care whilst also maximising value for money. The ways in which the government have attempted to secure these changes have been through the development of a strict regulatory, monitoring and performance assessment system that, by checking and making care practices visible and accountable, it is hoped will allow the achievement of positive outcomes. The aims are, of course, praiseworthy, but the evidence base to justify the approach is, as yet, weak. Indeed, meeting the standards and developing targets without investing them with a human and qualitative framework may detract from high-quality care as the achievement of targets becomes an end in itself.

Regulation, inspection and monitoring are not new methods and certainly began prior to the election of the Labour government of 1997. This can be seen in the regulatory framework for care homes in the 1980s mentioned earlier (see also Chapter 3). Also, the National Health Service and Community Care Act, 1990, implemented in April 1993, provided the backdrop for developing needs-driven assessments and arm's-length inspections, the creation of eligibility criteria and performance standards against which services could be measured and reported upon. The philosophical shift of the New Right to 'rolling back the frontiers of the State' (Friedman and Friedman, 1962; Talbot, 2001) have infiltrated welfare policies and even the change to New Labour and a 'third way' (Giddens 1998; Jordan, 2000) has continued to develop a market-oriented approach to care, whilst promoting ideas of quality that have been underpinned by performance management systems and target setting. The beginnings of the current performance and monitoring pathway are found in the social care White Paper *Modernising Social Services* (Department of Health, 1998b) which has informed the direction of social policy since. However, let's consider the wider picture of local government regulation and performance monitoring to set the context.

Best Value

Councils were given a duty to provide *best value* services under Part I of the Local Government Act, 1999. This duty requires councils to seek continuous improvement in all aspects of their service delivery through a fundamental methodology of Best Value Reviews, the aim of which was to ensure that local services are delivered to the highest standards and fully meet the needs of local residents whilst being good value for money. Later changes to the guidance issued have relaxed some of the requirements placed on those councils which are classed as 'excellent' or 'good' in their Comprehensive Performance Assessment (see below). But there is still a need for those councils to ensure that the delivery of local public services is of the highest quality. Originally, the Act asked for the development of a five-year programme of Best Value Review that was to be monitored and the results to be published annually in a Best Value Performance Plan which was to be seen in the context of other bureaucratic mechanisms within the council planning cycle, such as budget setting and community action plans.

Comprehensive Performance Assessment

The Audit Commission is an independent body responsible for ensuring that public monies are spent economically, effectively and efficiently in achieving high-quality local services for people. It operates a system of Comprehensive Performance Assessment (CPA), which was introduced in 2002, and is designed to assess the performance of councils and the services they provide with a view to highlighting areas in need of improvement. For example, in December 2005, the Audit Commission published the results of its comprehensive test (Audit Commission, 2005). The Commission found that over 70 per cent of councils were improving strongly or well, with 68 per cent achieving three- or four-star performance and five councils achieving the top category of assessment for both improvement and performance. However, alongside the very positive results, there were ten councils reported as not delivering services of an acceptable standard. The CPA uses other materials and monitoring reports produced by other bodies or for other purposes so as not to duplicate effort needlessly – for instance, the annual service assessments produced by the Commission for Social Care Inspection (CSCI) which cover children and young people's services and adult social care. The information collected feeds into the 'direction of travel' judgement and CPA star category. There are four labels that might be given to indicate how the council is faring overall. These are:

- Improving strongly
- Improving well

- Improving adequately
- Not improving adequately.

The CPA is a broad assessment, however, that doesn't necessarily reflect good work achieved in some council services in a council that might be underperforming in others. In respect of social services we need to consider the specific data collected under the performance assessment framework.

ACTIVITY 4.2

Search the website for a local authority CPA. Check the areas that may be relevant when considering adult protection issues and think about how this method of performance management may help in structuring and providing services and how it may hinder it.

Social Services Performance Assessment

The Performance Assessment Framework (PAF) represents the methodology designed to monitor the performance of all councils with social services responsibilities (CSSRs). From 2004, heralded by the Care Standards Act, 2000, the CSCI became the single body responsible for social care inspection and assumed responsibility for the administration and reporting about the PAF.

The PAF is operated in the context of Best Value and councils are expected to provide and deliver social services by the most effective, economic and efficient means available. The central aim is to secure continuous improvement and to demonstrate they have taken into account the four 'Cs':

- Challenge
- Compare
- Consult
- Compete.

Where councils fail to deliver Best Value, the government does have powers to intervene.

The PAF is a collection of data about nationally determined Performance Indicators (PIs) which, taken together, provide a view of how the council is serving its local people. The indicators are designed to cover as many aspects of social services as possible but to be still manageable in terms of completion. The PIs are separated into three sections covering children and families, adults and older people and management and resources and they are measured against five standards:

- National priorities and strategic objectives
- Cost and efficiency
- Effectiveness of service delivery and outcomes
- Quality of services for users and carers
- Fair access to services.

In December 2005, the CSCI published the seventh set of PAF indicators (CSCI, 2005a), and, as confirmed in the Audit Commission's CPAs, adult services appear to be improving. This general improvement in service provision is useful when considering vulnerability and protection issues – services seem to be responsive. The adult care PIs themselves cover residential and nursing home care, support at home, waiting times and care management issues such as reviews held. Although there are no specific or separate PIs concerning adult protection, an important aspect of performance assessment is the information reported on the protection of adults from abuse. The 2004–5 report stated that 145 (96.7 per cent) of councils have multi-agency adult protection procedures that are in place and operational and that 99 publish annual reports on vulnerable adult work (CSCI, 2005c).

ACTIVITY 4.3

Visit the CSCI website and look at some of the indicators for an authority you know. Repeat the task for the previous activity in respect of abuse and reporting.

Since 2005–6, the CSCI has been working with the Healthcare Commission and Audit Commission on a series of joint inspections into services for older people and how the NHS and local authorities are working together with partners to improve the lives of older people in general. A series of indicators is being developed with the aim of improving service provision for older people.

ACTIVITY 4.4

How might these indicators be used to support and enhance services which are aimed at protecting vulnerable adults? You may want to consider response times to adult protection procedures, service provision, reporting and monitoring and so on.

Monitoring the monitors (*Quis custodes custodiet?*)

There is great faith in the power of regulation to protect vulnerable individuals and to improve service provision and delivery. Indeed, those who are involved in regulation and inspection are also subject to the modernising agenda's emphasis on such practices, as can be seen in the CSCI (2005b) document *Inspecting for Better Lives – Delivering Change*.

The CSCI works at local, regional and national levels. Locally, it is responsible for registering private and voluntary care services, inspecting, assessing and reviewing all care services, even those run by the local council, and inspecting boarding schools, residential special schools and further education establishments with young people under eighteen years old attending. Any local inspection reports undertaken will be published and the local council will be provided with details of the numbers and the quality of private and voluntary care services in that area. If there are complaints about care service providers it is CSCI that will deal with them, and it will also review complaints made about social services. Its main methodology for assessing quality is by inspection, which may be announced or unannounced. Care provision is reviewed and inspected against National Minimum Standards. A judgement is made that the standard is·

- Exceeded (provision is commendable)
- Met (there being no shortfalls)
- Almost met (there were minor shortfalls)
- Not met (there were major shortfalls).

At a national level, the CSCI undertakes the following functions:

- drawing together national information about the state of social care
- informing policy-makers of the impact local and national policies are having on people
- reporting annually to Parliament on the state of social care
- carrying out research studies into social care
- commenting on social care research undertaken by other organisations.

All this sounds positive, and the reports indicate that improvements are being made. However, we need to accept that there remain serious concerns about quality of care as shown by media reports into care failures or mistakes (CSCI, 2006), which may indicate changing expectations and a continual desire to do better as this seems to be a consistent concern in countries with sophisticated care systems (see Proctor, 2002, for a US example). Moreover, we need to be alert to the concerns of Clough (1994), who notes that the regulation of social care may make people less trustworthy as service providers begin to rely on the regulators to impose the Standards rather than seeking improvement themselves.

Marshall (2006) critiques the ideology of performance management, recognising the change in direction from a rolling back of state provision to a reformed welfare system in which increased choice and user involvement characterise care practices (see Ham, 2006, in respect of the health service). Whilst he acknowledges some of the positive outcomes achieved in driving service priorities by assessing performance, Marshall is clear that the meeting of performance indicators privileges the meeting of broad aims and leaves out the needs of individuals or minority interests and may, at times, lead to case management to satisfy indicators rather than human need. Casey et al. (2005) consider that performance management is a mixed blessing, driving forward standards in some areas but presenting dangers of inconsistencies in practice and seeing performance management as a single event or end in itself. The importance of user perspectives is acknowledged in the performance indicators but these refer to quantitative measures of speed of service delivery and event occurrence, and not necessarily to what works best, to what is valued and to qualitative appreciation of services. Fairfax et al. (2005) report on the development of a monitoring tool for the Bradford Health Action Zone which shows that measures can be taken, but they recognise that this type of approach is still in its infancy. A more critical approach has been taken by Adcroft and Willis (2005), who suggest that existing performance management systems are more likely to commodify and deprofessionalise public sector services rather than improve them.

ACTIVITY 4.5

If you were wishing to include service user perspectives of performance of services into an evaluation, what questions do you think would be useful to ask in order to get as full a picture as possible of the service? Make a note of the likely areas that such questions would cover. You may also want to consider the differences between measures relating to service provision and perceptions about the value of services.

Individual quality assurance and enhancement

Individual practitioners are subject to monitoring by managers collecting data for performance management purposes. At times, this may seem somewhat removed from the demands of daily practice and to have little to offer individuals requiring social services. However, such monitoring aims to contribute to better service planning and provision, as we have seen, and, is, therefore, an important component of individual social care practice. Performance management and quality monitoring are not the end of the story; they concern services at the level of policy, management and overall planning, and we need to acknowledge ways in which individual social care practitioners can monitor and enhance the quality of their own practice.

The GSCC Code of Practice for Social Care Employees (GSCC, 2002) is clear in its promotion of best-quality work, keeping up to date and developing one's own approach to improving practice. For social workers, in particular, it is a prerequisite of re-registration that continued professional development is undertaken. Therefore, one way in which practitioners may contribute further to quality enhancement is in ensuring they are up to date with policy and legislative developments and research into effective practice. Training and development teams in some organisations and local authorities will be able to provide some courses aimed at updating both knowledge and practice. All training and development units are different, of course, with many local authority teams having a corporate rather than specific function and many smaller agencies concentrating on basic skills development.

However, it is a clear requirement for those working in situations in which there may be adult protection issues that training is undertaken in the local adult protection procedures. There are two lines of responsibility in ensuring this is done. It is the line manager's duty to plan for this training and to ensure that all staff complete it. It is, however, part of the individual social care professional's responsibility as part of his or her appraisal to be up to date and important that individuals plan for their own training and development needs. Clearly, undertaking training in the local adult protection procedure will not automatically ensure that people are better served or protected. There may also be those who suggest, somewhat cynically, that monitoring the completion of such courses is tokenistic, simply bureaucratic and undertaken as an end in itself. However, it does mean that local ways of working across agencies are more widely known and it provides individual practitioners with an important opportunity to update knowledge and explore issues of adult protection relevant to their work, not forgetting the professional responsibility that goes with such knowledge. In many instances, since such training is multi-agency with participants from a range of different organisations which all have an involvement in adult protection, it also provides practitioners with the chance to meet and exchange views about practice issues, roles and responsibilities with a wide variety of professionals from different agencies.

There is a further way in which practitioners can assure the quality of their work. Evidence-based practice as a concept has both its advocates and its critics, the latter often suggesting that the complexities and fluidities of human and social life proscribe the very idea of practice based on research evidence and that the development of 'practice wisdom' or an intuitive, indefinable approach based on experience is what is needed rather than evidence from quasi-scientific studies. Whilst the development of practice wisdom based on experience is not to be dismissed, it must be recognised that it is based on evidence gained from engagement in practice, internalised by professionals and used again because of the outcomes that are expected. What is important is that a practitioner identifies and articulates this evidence, becoming a research-minded practitioner who conducts his or her own evaluations of practice and builds a body of knowledge which informs his or her social care practice.

CASE STUDY 4.2: BUILDING KNOWLEDGE

When working as a specialist social worker in a team for people with dementia, one of us (Parker) used a single-case approach to evaluating interventions with older people experiencing stress in situations at risk of developing into abuse. Whilst the research literature is clear that stress is not a cause of abuse it has been found that the perceptions of how stressful a situation was led some people to take actions that were not always protective or helpful in preventing abuse (Steinmetz, 1990). By reducing the perceptions of stress and developing alternative strategies the risk of potential abuse was lessened (see Parker, 1998).

In adult protection work, as in other forms of social work and social care practice, it is important that individual practitioners evaluate, reflect on and theorise about their practice in order to provide the best possible services for those with whom they are working. It is also crucial that practitioners are aware of and able to apply the research of others concerning how best to work in protecting and supporting individuals in need of protection, with their families and carers, and in developing community responses to pertinent issues. By taking this responsibility as an individual each practitioner is involved in a kind of micro-level monitoring and performance management exercise. Whilst there might be a number of limitations and potential dangers with the existing performance management culture in social care, practitioners can work within it to ensure that the spirit behind it takes precedence rather than an unconsidered application of its letter.

SUMMARY

This chapter has provided an overview of monitoring, performance assessment and the reasoning behind it. As well as considering the importance of evaluating and improving services, the centrality of developing thoughtful, evidence-based practice in which workers develop their own understandings and add to the body of knowledge about 'what works' has also been described.

KEY READING

Butler, S. and Lymbery, M. (2004) *Social Work Ideals and Practice Realities*, Basingstoke: Macmillan.

Coulshed, V., Mullender, A., with Jones, D. and Thompson, N. (2006) *Management in Social Work* (3rd edition), Basingstoke: Palgrave.

Department of Health (2006a) *Our Health, Our Care, Our Say: A New Direction for Community Services*, London: Department of Health.

Harris, J. (2004) Consumerism: social development or social delimitation, *International Social Work*, 47, 4, 533–42.

Lavalette, M., Ferguson, I. and Mooney, G. (2002) *Rethinking Welfare: A Critical Perspective*, London: Sage.

CHAPTER 5

ASSESSMENT

OBJECTIVES

By the end of this chapter you should:

- understand the role of assessment in social care with vulnerable adults

- be able to describe some of the key elements of the assessment process

- be able to describe some of the particular aspects of assessments relating to the abuse of vulnerable adults

- be able to evaluate the function of assessment within the protection of vulnerable adults.

INTRODUCTION

In this chapter we emphasise the importance of conducting a comprehensive assessment as an essential part of the social and health care response to the abuse of vulnerable adults. Within social care and health practice, assessment is a key activity, which many people would identify as central to all practice (McDonald, 1999). There are philosophical debates concerning the purpose of assessment in social care that it is important to bear in mind. In a world in which assessment may be increasingly prescribed (Parker and Bradley, 2003; Parker, 2007a), it is easy to conceptualise assessment as an agency task. However, the overall aim of a social care assessment is to identify the particular needs of the individual and the issues that need to be worked on. It is an activity that should be conducted with the person rather than on the person, and this requires skills on the part of the practitioner in engaging the vulnerable adult to participate in the process as fully as possible (Smale et al., 2000; Milner and O'Byrne,

2002). Assessment also assists the practitioner in the development of a care plan that is suited to the individual and also, eventually, in deciding which interventions are most relevant. Of course, this is not necessarily a linear process from assessment through to intervention but is ongoing, giving the practitioner and service user a chance to monitor the appropriateness and effectiveness of the work (Parker, 2007a). We return to this later in the chapter. In the case of abuse of a vulnerable adult, it is necessary to consider which interventions may be needed in order to reduce further risk of abuse taking place. The roles of the social care practitioner within assessment include developing a relationship, making an assessment with the individual and working to develop an appropriate care plan that is tailored to meet individual needs. The role of the practitioner may also, in some instances, involve the provision of appropriate services, although this will depend on particular situations.

Social care practitioners in the UK work within the overall context of care management. Those workers practising as social workers or care managers have to work to the National Health Service and Community Care Act, 1990. It is in section 47 of this Act that the role of assessment is plainly stated. Community care assessment, undertaken by social workers, is a statutory duty but is also viewed as a service in its own right. If the assessment indicates a need for services then the decision to provide these services represents a separate duty. The exact form that the assessment should take is also left up to local authorities to decide. This has led, in some cases, to rather rigid assessments that are based on a single event and that use quite rigid criteria. As we have seen in Chapter 3, the relevant legislation states that there should be an assessment of the person's needs for services, followed by a decision concerning provision. This means that the assessment process itself is based on two stages. First there is the overall assessment of need, including needs for services. This is then followed by a decision about which service, if any will be provided. The decision about service provision depends on the rationing process established by that CSSR, which has been determined by the setting of local eligibility criteria. It is within this legislative context that social workers first come into contact with abuse of vulnerable adults and begin their assessments of the situation.

ACTIVITY 5.1

Imagine that your team has received a referral for a community care assessment of a person with complex health problems related to disability (not involving issues relating to protection). What areas of the individual's life and circumstances do you think should be covered by an assessment?

At the heart of any community care assessment undertaken within the remit of the Act is the concept of 'need'. This is a very difficult term to define satisfactorily. It is to a large extent left to each local council to agree on what this is in the light of their resources and policies. Because of some inconsistency from government between legislation and guidance, Mandelstam (1999) asks whether it is 'needs-for-services' or 'needs in the abstract' that should be assessed. When the change from an assessment for a particular service to needs-led assessment was introduced in 1993, when the Act was implemented, it was welcomed in principle by many social workers. However, as we have seen, the legislation talks about 'needs for services' rather than needs in the abstract (S.47 1 a). In addition to this, questions of eligibility criteria further complicate the matter as to who may actually receive a service. Also principles of fairness and equity might demand that assessment takes into account all the services available and the extent of resources so as to enable full participation in the assessment by the person. This begins to address some of the requirements of developing an exchange relationship that values the person as an expert in their own right rather than a procedural or simple questioning approach used by the practitioner without including the service user (Smale et al., 2000).

Using an assessment to obtain a full picture of a situation, to discover the impact of the circumstances on those involved and the wants, needs and wishes of individuals involved, it is then possible to plan, develop and implement interventions that will result in change for the individual and their situation. It is also possible, where necessary, to protect them from (further) situations of abuse.

ACTIVITY 5.2

Now imagine that your team has received a referral for a community care assessment of a complex situation relating to a vulnerable adult (this time involving issues relating to protection). What areas of the individual's life and circumstances do you think should be covered by an assessment? Are there different areas that you can think of that ought to be covered and included in the assessment?

Undertaking an holistic assessment, covering all aspects of the individual's life can be a time-consuming process. This may particularly be the case if this requires collecting information from other significant people from the individual's network in order to really find out about the person's views and wishes. At the most basic level of assessment, Sutton (1994) has suggested that there are four key areas which need to be included as the key elements of the assessment process. These are:

- What are the main concerns, issues, problems or needs?
- What are the priority areas?
- Who are the key parties involved?
- Why have the difficulties developed?

A further question relates to the timing of the referral or the concern (why has this happened now?); this can be particularly useful when considering situations that have evidently been ongoing and developing for some time and when it might be useful to know what has led to the referral being made at that particular point in time. Although these key areas clearly apply to all care assessments that practitioners are involved in, they can clearly be adapted for use in the assessment of situations of possible abuse. If we look at a range of models of social care assessment, we find the following characteristics as outlined by Parker (2007a):

- preparation, planning and engagement
- information collection and creating a problem profile
- preliminary analysis
- testing hypotheses and deeper analysis
- use of the information collected, and creation of a (safety) plan.

GUIDANCE ON PROTECTION POLICIES AND PROCEDURES

The Department of Health guidance on developing policies and procedures provides some of the steps that are needed towards protecting vulnerable adults from abuse (Department of Health, 2000a). It is still reactive in many ways and considers ways in which people can be protected from further abuse or indeed how to work when abuse has already happened or has been alleged to have taken place. The document, *No Secrets*, has section seven status under the Local Authority Social Services Act, 1970. This means that it must be complied with in all but exceptional circumstances although it is not law. The guidance requires councils with social services responsibilities (CSSRs) to take the lead role in the co-ordination of responses to issues relating to adult protection, for example when an allegation of abuse is made. It does not, however, mean that CSSRs always have to take the overall lead in adult protection and be in charge of all investigations and assessments of abuse, although the distinction is in some ways quite subtle. CSSRs have the task of ensuring that policies and procedures are in place at local levels on a multi-agency basis and that there are processes that will be followed when an allegation is made. However, the guidance does not mandate all other organisations to be involved in the process, although this is indicated as good practice in the document. This means that at times other organisations may have other priorities and may not be involved in situations of adult protection even though this might be advisable.

For people working within social care and care settings this guidance is central. Whilst it covers more than care or institutional settings, it makes multi-agency working an imperative in all settings. The guidance was introduced in March 2000 and implemented in October 2001, and Social Services Departments (now CSSRs) were charged with the lead co-ordinating role in responding to the abuse of vulnerable adults (and, as we have seen above, in ensuring that multidisciplinary responses to adult protection have developed in local areas). For these reasons we include an extended section concerning this guidance.

The key aim of the guidance is to create a framework for action in which agencies will work together to prevent or respond to the abuse of adults. In developing these local frameworks, service users, carers and representative groups need to be consulted. The document itself provides a structure for developing coherent multi-agency policies and procedures.

Assessment and *No Secrets*

Whilst issues concerning definitions of abuse are dealt with in the document, as we saw in Chapter 2, the main thrust of this guidance document concerns administrative policies and the development of inter-agency policies, operational policies, procedures and guidance for staff, service users, carers and the general public. However, it is not simply administrative measures that are promoted. Skills for effective practice are considered to be paramount. Assessment processes and the skills associated with good assessment practice are central. Whatever policies and procedures are designed and implemented in each locality, staff must have well developed skills in assessment as well as an open mind about the allegations that have been made. Indeed, *No Secrets* states the following objectives for an adult protection investigation:

- to establish facts
- to assess the needs of the vulnerable adult for protection, support and redress and
- to make decisions with regard to what follow-up action should be taken with regard to the perpetrator and the service or its management if they have been culpable, ineffective or negligent.

(Department of Health, 2000a, para. 6.19)

The document indicates that the principal priority at all times should be the safety and protection of the vulnerable adult. It is therefore stated that it is the responsibility of all staff (from whatever agency) to take action on any concern, suspicion or evidence of either abuse or neglect which relates to a vulnerable adult. The first action to take should therefore normally be to pass on those concerns either to a responsible agency or to an individual (preferably named) person within that agency so that an investigation can be planned and then undertaken if or as necessary.

There are a number of separate stages to any investigation of an adult protection matter. The document suggests that these are:

- reporting or referral made to a single initial point of contact
- precisely recording the factual details of the alleged or suspected abuse (this requires attention and sensitivity towards the vulnerable adult by the person taking down this information)
- an initial co-ordination of the process, which involves representation from all agencies that might have a role in the investigation or processes involved (this is sometimes referred to as a Strategy Meeting or Strategy Discussion)
- carrying out the investigation within the framework that has been jointly agreed at local level, in order to establish the facts of the case and
- decision-making in order to adequately protect the vulnerable adult, which could be at a meeting such as a case conference.

As can be seen above, one of the main differences between a Strategy Meeting and the case conference is really that of timing. Strategy Meetings are usually held before the full investigation starts (or as it is starting), partly in order to plan aspects of the process, and the case conference is held after the investigation has been completed. It therefore discusses the results of the investigation in order to establish what interventions or further actions are needed, such as the construction of a safety plan for the individual, including any services that might need to be provided within the care plan.

Once the facts surrounding the situation have been established, an assessment of need is likely to be necessary (unless the allegation is not proven). This assessment will require discussions, decisions and safety planning on a joint basis by all the agencies involved with the individual. It may therefore be the case that multiple agencies are not involved in separate assessments of need, but perhaps a joint assessment will be conducted by several practitioners from different disciplines, or with contributions from a number of different disciplines, in order to provide an holistic view of the individual and their circumstances. In addition, the following issues are stated as being important to consider within all assessments relating to adult protection:

- the vulnerability of the person
- the nature and extent of abuse
- the duration of abuse
- the impact(s) on the individual
- the risk of repetition or increasing seriousness.

This leads to the need for a number of questions in order to determine whether the person is suffering harm or exploitation, the level of risk(s) they are exposed to and whether they have the capacity to make their own decisions about risk and safety, whether they meet the eligibility criteria for the National Health Service and Community Care Act, 1990, and whether and what sort of intervention is in the individual's interests. The length of time that the alleged abuse has been occurring, and whether this is part of a pattern of abuse, is also relevant in relation to this, as in many situations it is unusual to come across just one single incident of abuse. In the last point above, it is also necessary for there to be some consideration of whether other vulnerable adults might be at risk of abuse as well as the individual concerned, as there may be additional risks to other service users in some settings (for example day care settings as well as care homes).

The assessment process is set out in procedural terms. However, social care practitioners should focus on the people involved and engage them in an exchange relationship that privileges, values and clearly includes the perspectives of those concerned (Smale et al., 2000; Parker, 2007a). The assessment should also focus not just on the impact of the alleged abuse on the person concerned but also on the depth of feelings of the person alleging the abuse. This is also important for practitioners working in care settings. In order to consider the impact as perceived by the individual, the practitioner must 'stand in the shoes of' the person making the allegation. This demands the development of empathic skills and an understanding of crisis theory and intervention, and gives credence to the growing interest in individual biographies and narratives (Milner and O'Byrne, 2002). Thus aspects of the guidance are clear in promoting an effective practitioner response to individual allegations of abuse. However, the guidance also concerns the systems in which social and health care are practised and emphasises the importance of working together across the different organisations involved in work with vulnerable adults.

In terms of the outcomes of the investigation and assessment, *No Secrets* indicates that an agreed action plan should be put together at the meeting convened to receive the assessment findings and plan for future safety needs; this meeting is often referred to as the case conference (Department of Health, 2000a). This plan should be included as part of the individual's care plan. The relevant agencies must then take appropriate steps to implement the action or safety plan. The plan should set out:

• what steps need to be taken to ensure the future safety of the individual
• what treatment or therapy might be required and accessed by the vulnerable adult
• what modifications, if any, are needed to service provision (for instance a change of placement, or the provision of carers of the same gender)
• what support is likely to be needed by the individual concerning any legal action that might be taken (either by the vulnerable adult or on their behalf, e.g. prosecution of the perpetrator of the abuse)
• what ongoing strategy for risk management might be necessary to assist and support the individual.

ASSESSMENT: RIGHTS AND RISKS

It has been acknowledged for some time now by both social work and health care practitioners that assessment is a dynamic and ongoing process and does not (or should not) just consist of the production of a one-off report at one particular point in time (Parker and Bradley, 2003; Coulshed and Orme, 2006). Assessments may take some time to carry out and complete, especially in relation to complex situations, and the practitioner has to be prepared for this to be the case. Additionally, practitioners need to be aware that in some ways an assessment is never fully completed given how quickly many interpersonal situations can change. Therefore there may be an almost continual need to re-assess the individual's needs as situations develop and alter. And as became apparent above, within the assessment process there are in any case a number of factors that need to be taken into account. This includes such factors as the risks of harm that the individual is exposed to, together with the risks that they may be able to manage themselves. Such issues as these have to be carefully considered and taken into account. This may be so for most, if not all, assessments, but perhaps especially when working with vulnerable adults.

In connection with these aspects, the rights of the individual to take risks and to take decisions also have to be appropriately assessed, perhaps especially in relation to issues relating to the individual's capacity to take decisions and to achieve informed consent. This requires, for instance that the individual is made aware of the potential risks involved with a particular action or actions and the possible consequences of taking a particular decision and is able to understand and make an informed choice about whether to take the risk or not. The guidance document is explicit that the capacity of the individual to take decisions about the arrangements relating to both any investigation and the management of the abusive situation needs to be taken into account. The following information is provided in relation to capacity:

> The vulnerable adult's capacity is the key to action since if someone has 'capacity' and declines assistance this limits the help that he or she may be given. It will not however limit the action that may be required to protect others who are at risk of harm. In order to make sound decisions, the

vulnerable adult's emotional, physical, intellectual and mental capacity in relation to self-determination and consent and any intimidation, misuse of authority or undue influence will have to be assessed.

(Department of Health, 2000a, para. 6.21)

As we have seen in Chapter 3 and will see later in chapters concerning both learning disability and mental health, the implementation of the Mental Capacity Act, 2005, from April 2007 will provide some much needed changes and safeguards relating to adults who lack capacity and the ability to take decisions.

ASSESSMENT AND ABUSE

As we have already seen, there are some factors that need to be given particular attention in relation to situations of abuse and vulnerability. Assessment of particular abusive situations should be 'needs-led but abuse focused' (Bennett et al., 1997, p. 173) so that, although the assessment is carried out within community care legislation and is holistic, covering all aspects of an individual's life and circumstances, a particular focus on abuse and the abusive situation may be absolutely essential within the assessment process in order to gain as complete an understanding as possible of the circumstances. In respect of values, it is fundamental that practitioners seek to develop a relationship built on trust and respect; this should be an exchange relationship that includes the person in the assessment and is built on mutuality as far as possible.

Within the assessment process, early guidance produced by government in relation to elder abuse (Department of Health, 1995) suggested that there were a number of questions that it could be helpful to include in an assessment, particularly when considering situations of alleged, potential or likely abuse. Although these questions were originally devised in relation to older people, as will be seen below, they could be adapted for use with other vulnerable adults. These questions appear in Box 5.1 and may be seen to offer the practitioner a useful framework and initial structure from which to further develop the assessment, as it is possible to see that a number of follow-up questions may arise from each of the major questions asked. This will help to ensure that the assessment can cover the ground that it needs to. From a thorough attention to detail during the information-gathering process, including the accurate recording of information provided in the answers to the questions asked, an assessment can be successfully completed.

BOX 5.1   ASSESSMENT QUESTIONS

Where do concerns arise from?
Why are they being raised now?
What action (if any) does the referrer expect to happen?
Does the vulnerable person or carer know about the referral and the concern?

Is there a need for an advocate for the older person?
What will be the likely outcome if assistance is refused?
What safeguards need to be established within the situation?

(Department of Health, 1995)

We have previously described processes of assessment that should be worked through in relation to abuse and vulnerability (Penhale et al., 2000). These include the following:

- Engage the client in the process and establish a relationship.
- Seek the client's views and offer choices.
- Negotiation and participation: emphasise values and choice.
- Explore the relationships between key people.
- Explore risks and dangerousness.
- Use assessment information to develop the care plan.
- Establish a safety plan if or as necessary.

Clearly the involvement of the individual in the process of assessment or investigation is of the essence here. Practitioners therefore need to have skills in engaging with service users and in enabling and facilitating involvement in processes and decisions (Warren, 2007). In many cases a comprehensive assessment of the situation will be necessary and this is multi-faceted, covering a wide range of different areas. It may also mean that there is a specific need to get the individual's views about the situation. The person should be offered the chance to have a separate interview and discussion with the practitioner. This will help to identify and clarify the individual's views and wishes. Some people may hold a view that it is always essential to see the individual on their own, apart from any carer or other person involved in the situation and that this is particularly important where situations of potential abuse are involved. However, although this may be desired, it may not always be possible to attain, perhaps particularly if the individual does not wish to be interviewed on their own, or for example may lack particular communication skills that may require a particular other person to be present to assist with the discussion. Where possible, the person should be given the choice to have a separate interview, however. It may also generally be quite fitting to make the same offer of a separate, private discussion to others involved in the situation and this may include the person who is considered to have been responsible for the abuse. It is important here that there are sufficient considerations by the practitioner before any such interview about the levels of risk, dangerousness and personal safety that may be present in such interviews. The decision that is reached about this must be an informed choice, shared with managers, which takes into account the desirability (or otherwise) of such actions.

It may also be the case, of course, that neither the vulnerable adult nor perhaps more particularly the alleged perpetrator should be interviewed separately by the practitioner if there is likely to be any police involvement in connection with a possible crime having been committed, as to hold such an interview may well compromise and prejudice any further inquiry by the police. This of course is likely to be a different situation from the initial process of obtaining basic information from the vulnerable adult about what has happened (which can be written down as they have said it).

However, in order to gain the maximum amount of information about an individual's situation, including knowledge about the relationship between the individuals involved, generally an interview of the individuals involved in the situation together is also necessary. Such an interview will help by providing information about the nature and quality of the relationship as well as the type and amount of interaction between the different individuals involved. This may also entail some degree of risk and danger, however, both for the vulnerable adult and also perhaps for the practitioner. Therefore, it is necessary to try to establish beforehand the degree of potential risk and dangerousness in holding a joint interview. So the related issues of individual safety for the older person and also for the practitioner need to be carefully considered. Within a potentially dangerous situation it may be wise to have two practitioners, or a practitioner and line manager, to try to ensure adequate protection for the individuals concerned. In such situations careful planning of the assessment process ahead of the event is needed and help from a specialist practitioner or consultant or line manager may be advisable.

CASE STUDY 5.1: WINIFRED AND EDWARD

A referral received in a social work office concerned an elderly lady, Mrs Winifred Downs, and her husband, Edward, who had moderately severe dementia. The neighbour who had made the referral was very concerned about the risk of harm to the lady and increasing threats that her husband had been heard making about and to his wife in recent weeks. As neither Mr nor Mrs Downs had previously been known to social services, the social worker decided to discuss the referral with her line manager. The team manager and social worker decided to contact the couple's GP for some further information about the situation. The doctor said that in his view Mr Downs was quite a dominant and powerful person, who had previously held quite a high rank in the Army, but the doctor did not think that Mr Downs would necessarily pose a major risk to outsiders, provided he was 'carefully handled'.

Since this information suggested some degree of unpredictability and risk, a decision was taken that a joint home visit to the couple would be made in order to try and involve both Mr and Mrs Downs in the assessment. This would also include attempts to interview each of them individually. The team manager decided to visit with the social worker as the other person involved. It was planned that concerns would be presented to the couple in a way that tried to achieve solutions and included both members of the couple as far as possible in both the assessment process and any subsequent care planning that took place.

As a result of the information gathered in the assessment, the practitioner must also consider some further issues of risk, such as whether the person involved poses a danger to themselves or others either by their actions or by a lack of actions. In order to form an opinion on the potential risk to self and others, the practitioner needs to take into account:

- how reliable the evidence about the risk is
- relevant past history including behaviour patterns
- the nature, extent and degree of likely risk
- how far any carers are willing and able to cope with the individual
- any misunderstandings about behaviour or intent that might occur as a result of assumptions based on gender, social and cultural background, ethnic origin and other medical or health conditions including deafness and other sensory impairments.

A number of inquiries into mental health tragedies recommend that accurate details of any violent incidents be maintained in an individual's case records (Stanley et al., 1999). The need for clear, concise but accurate and precise recording is absolutely necessary here. Violent incidents do not just refer to acts committed by an individual, and acts of violence directed towards a person also need to be documented. So although the vulnerable person may not himself or herself pose any risk of violence, the risk to them from others needs to be accurately documented as well as any risk to others involved. This would include, for example, the risk of violence directed towards care workers and other professionals involved. Such issues must be taken into account and fully documented. Additionally, relevant information about whether the situation has been positively substantiated, and if so, by whom, or whether it remains at the level of an allegation should also be detailed. It is also important that the views of the individuals involved are recorded. As far as possible, this should include the individuals' views concerning the violence or abuse, the abusive situation and what they think should happen about the situation.

Many CSSRs have been developing policies and procedures concerning the assessment and management of risk and dangerousness in recent years, as well as policies and procedures on responding to the abuse of vulnerable adults. Any actions taken by a practitioner should, of course, be in accordance with any such relevant guidelines or procedures that exist within a department. This may require that any decision is shared between a number of individuals, rather than taken by one individual on their own.

Using assessment knowledge to plan

As part of the assessment process an important element is to try to establish the principal cause of the abuse so that appropriate interventions can be offered within the care plan. So for example, if the abuse is principally due to the stress to a carer from looking after a person with complex needs, then the provision of services within the community may be appropriate in order to support, alleviate and monitor the situation. If, however, the abuse results from some psychopathology of the abuser, then an approach that provides for treatment of the abuser (for example, treatment for substance misuse) is likely to be preferable. However, even within such situations, some consideration of the needs of the vulnerable person for safety and protection is also likely to be necessary.

How willing the individuals are to engage in assessment and intervention is clearly fundamental in this context. If the practitioner can negotiate the boundary between the private and public worlds of individuals satisfactorily, then it is far more likely that the outcome of the intervention as well as the assessment will be positive. Obviously, if the person is willing to participate in assessment and any subsequent intervention in order to solve a problem then the outcome is far more likely to be successful. Not surprisingly, it is necessary to recognise the range and diversity of family forms and different cultural values and practices within both assessment and intervention practices in order to resolve the abusive situation and stop abuse from continuing.

Theory and skills

Despite what the Minister for Health implied when introducing the new degree in social work, theoretical knowledge and understanding are a prerequisite for good and effective practice and the deployment of skills. The Minister stated:

> Social work is a very practical job. It is about protecting people and changing their lives, not about being able to give a fluent and theoretical explanation of why they got into difficulties in the first place.
>
> (Smith, 2002)

Social work and social care work are indeed very practical, but being practical involves knowing why something might be happening and what might be done to produce change in that particular situation. It also requires the research-mindedness to apply knowledge to protect vulnerable service users, no matter what the setting (Parker and Bradley, 2003).

Social workers and social care practitioners are well versed in working creatively and flexibly with individuals and groups of people. Often, it seems to be the case that practitioners hide these talents or doubt their abilities. It is certainly true that many deny that they use models or theories in practice, although they do work in ways that demonstrate using theories (Howe, 1998); they are systematic, based on prior experience of what has worked in similar situations before, and often implicitly use tried and tested models. It is important, however, that social work and social care practitioners should develop evidence-based practice that clearly demonstrates what they are doing and why this is the case. In working with individuals who are abused or vulnerable and those who abuse, social workers need to develop a repertoire of practice skills and knowledge that can be translated and used across a range of practice settings.

Clearly, good interpersonal skills are central to effective social care practice in care settings. Whilst we can identify core skills in active listening we must be mindful of subtle cultural differences in the ways in which these skills are deployed. Interpersonal skills and listening may help when working with a person who has experienced abuse. They may need more in-depth and professional counselling. It may be that they need to learn new skills, develop assertiveness and increase confidence. These may also be needed for people who abuse. However, challenging and disputing and working together to manage behaviours are important individual techniques here. Grounding in cognitive behavioural approaches is important for those working with vulnerable adults who abuse. These models rely on identifying triggers and prompts to behaviour in certain settings, at certain times or reactions to events. They also rely on identifying factors in the person's environment that maintain or make more likely that behaviour in the future: what does the person get from acting in this way that they do not get from elsewhere (Parker, 1998)?

The following case study develops the use of a helpful cognitive behavioural model for managing anger in a man whose impulse control was lowered. It must be stated that not all abuse is physical, that causal factors are complex, and to address issues fully necessitates reviewing all systems within care settings. However, these models form part of an effective array of helping tools for working with people who abuse.

CASE STUDY 5.2: JEREMY

Jeremy Jones attends a resource centre for people with learning disabilities. Jeremy is well liked by staff and other members and takes an active part in the activities run by the centre. However, Jeremy has a tendency to hit out at the nearest person whenever something goes wrong for him or when he does not get his own way. For many years this behaviour has been tolerated as simply the way Jeremy deals with frustration. A new manager has determined that Jeremy needs to learn more appropriate ways of expressing frustration or annoyance. Things came to a head recently, when he hit a female member of staff and cracked her tooth. He was suspended from the day centre for a week.

The social worker, Mark, looked with staff at the times Jeremy became angry and spent time with Jeremy looking at things that made him angry. Mark thought it possible that Jeremy could examine what happened 'inside' when he became angry. Jeremy and Mark spent time getting to know one another and began exploring the feelings and physical sensations that developed when Jeremy became angry. They then began to identify points in this process at which Jeremy felt he had no other option but to get angry and hit out. This allowed them to search for alternative ways of bringing his anger to the attention of staff before Jeremy felt out of control. Jeremy enjoyed this process and was able to check his anger. The process worked, however, because all the staff were party to it. If the work had been done in isolation from others at the day centre, the response to Jeremy's anger would have been different and could possibly have lead to further incidents of violence.

Some of the dangers inherent in using a cognitive-behavioural approach or indeed any other approach centre on a lack of training or lack of consistency across practitioners or even within the agency. There are clear training and supervisory implications for intervening to protect or to enhance the skills of people worked with in care settings. It must always be remembered that the effects of abuse can be increased if intervention techniques and strategies are used incorrectly or inappropriately, and the need for intervention and which form of intervention should be used must be carefully considered. The use of inappropriate interventions may of course even constitute abuse in its own right.

SUMMARY

In this chapter we have explored the need for a comprehensive assessment in order to take into account the views and wishes of all relevant parties but perhaps particularly the vulnerable person who is the focus of the assessment. Participation in assessment is fundamental here. The value base of social and health work is fundamental to good assessment practice. Also, in assessing abuse of vulnerable adults, risk assessment and risk management need to be taken into account. This requires a co-ordinated response and one that is multidisciplinary in nature.

There are many different and varied approaches to assessment of possible situations of adult abuse. This is in part due to the fact that there are many different types of abuse and a wide range of vulnerabilities and adults at risk of abusive situations. The actual method of assessment that is used will of course depend on the overall context, the role and function of the practitioner, and any agency requirements. Whatever approach is taken, it is essential that practitioners recognise that the purpose of assessment is to gain a full picture of a situation, the impact of elements of the situation on those involved and the wants, wishes and needs of individuals affected. This is necessary so that the practitioner can then appropriately plan, develop and implement interventions that will result in change. In the next chapter we will consider ways in which practitioners can work with vulnerable adults who have been abused and those who abuse.

KEY READING

Parker, J. (2007a) The process of social work: assessment, planning, intervention and review. In M. Lymbery and K. Postle (eds) *Social Work: A Companion to Learning*, London: Sage.
Smale, G., Tucson, G. and Statham, D. (2000) *Social Work and Social Problems*, Basingstoke: Macmillan.
Warren, J. (2007) *Social Work and Service Users*, Exeter: Learning Matters.

CHAPTER 6

VULNERABILITY, RISK AND ABUSE

OBJECTIVES

By the end of this chapter you should:

- be able to describe core elements of interventions relating to protection from abuse and harm

- understand the place of multi-agency work in protecting vulnerable adults

- be able to consider some of the benefits and limitations of particular types of interventions

- be able to evaluate the function of guidance to prevent or limit risks or to deal with abuse and harm that have taken place.

INTRODUCTION

This chapter takes a multi-level and multi-dimension approach to working effectively to reduce and counter abuse. In essence, this means we consider legislation and social policy issues which are relevant to developing positive long-term strategies to counteract abuse wherever this occurs (in the domestic arena or in care settings). There is a consideration of local and regional policy initiatives, procedural issues developed across organisations and agencies and within teams. Within this discussion, the importance of partnership and multidisciplinary working between the different agencies involved is emphasised. The limitations of care management approaches and the centrality of risk assessment or risk management approaches is critiqued.

Initially, the typology of different aspects and attributes of abuse which was outlined in Chapter 2 is used and extended in order to develop our understanding of the relative effectiveness and importance of strategies and intervention techniques.

The levels or dimensions of abuse can be referred to as micro level (individual), mezzo level (community or agency) and macro level (structural or societal) (Bennett et al., 1997). Acknowledging that abuse can occur at personal, community or societal levels illustrates once again that there are many different forms of abuse and neglect and that the spectrum of abuse is really quite broad. This is especially the case in respect of working with abuse in care settings, as shown in Table 6.1. This shows the abuse perpetrated by people working in social care settings or by the regimes themselves together with possible interventions that can occur at the different levels mentioned above.

Table 6.1 does not deal with abuse perpetrated by other users of care settings or by relatives and acquaintances of the abused person, although as we have seen in previous chapters this does undoubtedly occur. We must also remember that social care practitioners can be most effective in working in these situations. Interventions in this type of situation would appear as in Table 6.2.

Discrimination against people because of certain characteristics they possess or do not possess, because of social divisions, categorisations and shared assumptions by those holding greater power or influence are widespread throughout society. Before we examine policy, procedure and personal practice we need to consider some of the ways in which discrimination abuses individuals at a range of different levels and ways. Whilst there has been a backlash against some of the excesses of so-called 'political correctness', social care practitioners deal on a daily basis with people who are exploited or made vulnerable as a result of discrimination, oppression and exclusion (Parker, 2007b). As we saw in Chapter 2, one of the key challenges for social care practitioners working in care settings is to recognise that the settings themselves, the care practices which

Table 6.1 Intervention types: abuse by care workers

Types of abuse	Macro level – political/structural	Mezzo level – community/agency	Micro level – individual
Abuse of vulnerable adults by professionals and care staff in care settings	Public Interest Disclosure Act, 1998 (whistle-blowing), Care Standards Act, 2000, Registered Homes Act, 1984 (amended 1991)	Increased participation in care settings by members of local communities will produce more 'open' environment and increased chance of abuse being detected	Supervision, training, support about recognising and dealing with abuse
Abuse in care settings (abusive regimes)	Care Standards Act, 2000, GSCC Code of Practice for Employers, Government guidance and regulation (e.g. minimum standards for care homes; 'Home Life' and 'A Better Home Life')	Increased participation in care settings by members of local communities will produce more 'open' environment and increased chance of abuse being detected	Individual responsibility to identify and report abusive practices; assisted by supervision, support and training

Source: adapted from Bennett et al. (1997, p. 10).

Table 6.2 Intervention types: abuse by relatives

Types of abuse	Macro level – political/structural	Mezzo level – community/agency	Micro level – individual
Abuse of vulnerable adults by relatives in care settings	Use of Adult Protection procedures at local levels. Use of appropriate legislation, where necessary (e.g. Theft Act, 1968)	Increased participation in care settings by members of local communities will produce more 'open' environment and increased monitoring of situations	Information, awareness raising about abuse support and review or monitoring of the situation and the individuals involved
Abuse of vulnerable adults by relatives in domestic or community settings	Use of Adult Protection procedures at local levels and development of safety plans for individuals. Use of appropriate legislation, where necessary (e.g. Theft Act, 1968)	Increased participation by members of local communities in their local communities and with those who are vulnerable will produce an increased chance of abuse being detected	Individual responsibility to identify and report abuse; assisted by information, public and professional awareness raising so that abuse is detected and dealt with

Source: adapted from Bennett et al. (1997, p. 10).

underpin them and social care staff as a group can all discriminate and oppress individuals and, at times, act abusively towards them. Subsequent to this recognition is the acknowledgement of a need to change this situation and also to seek effective ways of working with individuals, with diversity and in non-discriminatory ways.

How can this be done? Just as there are many different settings in which practitioners may encounter service users who are vulnerable, there are many different forms and levels of discrimination and oppression, which may lead to exclusion (see also Chapter 10). Being open to the view that discrimination exists and that we may all contribute to its maintenance in some way is a first step to being able to challenge and alter it. The converse may also be true. To claim that one never discriminated but was also anti-discriminatory may deflect from acknowledging the complex nature of discrimination and oppression and the possibility that we may all contribute to it. It is also important for practitioners to acknowledge the range of strategies that can be used to counteract such discrimination.

At the policy and procedural level, care agencies have a responsibility to develop and implement anti-harassment and equal opportunities policies. This is important in two respects. First, staff need to know that they are valued and will be treated with respect and, second, service users need to be assured that care services and access to them will be fair, and not provided discriminately on the basis of health status, gender, age, ethnicity or belief. This will involve training for staff, not just concerning the content of these policies and procedures but also in terms of shifting the culture of care to one that is inclusive of all (within the remit of the agency). This will probably also require some shift in attitudes and beliefs in order to achieve cultural and organisational change(s).

These central changes in both the culture and practice of organisations will be more likely to come about if staff are afforded regular supportive and developmental supervision. In an increasingly managerial and performance-related environment, supervision has become, at times, synonymous with managerial accountability. It is a system in which cases are checked, procedures are seen to be followed and initiatives are audited. Of course, it is important to be able to assure employers and indeed the public that work has been completed according to guidelines and procedures and that standards are upheld. This is not the sole reason for supervision, however, as supervision should also be used for professional and developmental purposes (Tsui, 2005). It is also important as a way to value staff by supportive and developmental approaches that reflect a practice culture of respect, valuing people and a concern for best practice. Support for staff who are working with vulnerable individuals, including those who are facing abuse or abusive situations where there are no instant solutions is clearly very important in order to assist those staff to work effectively in such circumstances.

In Chapter 1 we introduced the GSCC Codes of Practice and the BASW Code of Ethics that social workers and social care workers now have to work to. These codes are important tools in facilitating anti-discriminatory practice. It is important that an anti-discriminatory focus permeates all levels of care practice: policy, agency procedure and individual practice. As social work and social care move towards greater regulation, codes of practice and ethics can guide both supervision and practice. They may be particularly useful in identifying aspects of practice that are in need of further attention and development.

The following two case studies portray some aspects of discrimination in social care settings and how it was dealt with.

CASE STUDY 6.1: MELINDA

Melinda Bryan was living with her mother, who had become very forgetful. For two years this situation got worse, with Melinda and her mother being told by the doctor that there was little he could do and it was 'just old age'. Melinda sought further advice and, after changing her doctor, her mother was diagnosed as having Alzheimer's disease. Melinda did not know much about Alzheimer's disease and sought information but found that few people were willing to offer advice. Eventually she tried to get some relief from the daily caring but was told by a social worker that she was doing a good job looking after her mother and it would be inappropriate to send in someone her mother did not know so it would be best if she continued to look after her fully.

CASE STUDY 6.2: TESSA

Tessa Lockington was a student social worker visiting a man in a sheltered housing complex. She visited with the warden of the complex who, after knocking once on the man's door, opened it before there was any answer from inside and walked in. Tessa asked, 'I'm new to this but do you always walk into the residents' accommodation without waiting for an answer?'

In the first example, Melinda was let down by the services she was seeking help from and her vulnerability was increased by the lack of information available and lack of support offered. In the second, Tessa showed clearly her recognition of the inappropriateness of the warden's actions and challenged the warden in a gentle but clear manner.

Just as policies and procedures can contribute to discrimination and oppression in social care settings, they can be used as a powerful force for effective protection and for guiding practices designed to combat abuse. In section 6 of the Department of Health (2000a) guidance on developing policies and procedures for working with abuse and adult protection, the procedures most likely to affect practitioners in care settings are detailed. It also concerns the responses to be made in individual cases. As we saw in Chapter 5, the principal priority is always to ensure the safety and protection of vulnerable adults. All staff, therefore, have a duty to pass on information regarding abuse or neglect so that it is investigated appropriately (see also the Public Interest Disclosure Act, 1998, as discussed in Chapter 3).

If staff are uncertain or unclear about what they should do and do not feel that they can discuss this with a line manager, for example if the manager is implicated in the situation, they should make contact with an organisation such as Action on Elder Abuse or Public Concern at Work in order to discuss the options and processes further. Both of these voluntary organisations can provide advice and information to people. The latter organisation has specialised for some years now in providing support to people who wish to 'whistle-blow' from many different sectors of employment but they have built up some expertise in assisting practitioners from the health and social care sectors and supporting people through the processes involved, if necessary.

The Department of Health (2000a, para. 6.4) guidance is clear that intervention that is agreed upon with the individual service user may be therapeutic, supportive, disciplinary or criminal in its nature or intent. Any investigation will therefore seek to achieve the following objectives:

- Establish the facts.
- Assess needs for protection and support.
- Make decisions about follow-up action with all involved.

All procedures developed will contain a statement outlining roles, responsibilities, authority and accountability for the individuals involved. They will also detail such operational matters as what to do when an allegation is received, what to do in emergencies and what to do when procedures are not followed. They will set out information on recording, collecting data, communication and information sharing between agencies and contact details for resources and experts. Procedures may well include protocols on specific areas such as confidentiality or information sharing between agencies.

Practical advice is also presented within procedures in relation to support for the person making the allegation and perhaps also their family, to preserving confidentiality where possible, to fairness, protection and support for those involved, including at times practitioners. The different stages involved in the investigation are presented, which usually includes all those involved reporting to a single point or reference, recording being precise and sensitive. The investigation should be co-ordinated and carried out in accordance with a jointly agreed framework. Decisions should be recorded using shared forms and records of all incidents should be kept. This raises training and practice issues for practitioners in social care settings and raises the questions: what should be recorded and when may rights to confidentiality be breached? It is also important to be confident that the information recorded can be easily used to collect statistical information, as this may help agencies protect adults more effectively in the future. This demands that social care practitioners recognise the centrality of recording in their practice.

BOX 6.1 NORFOLK ADULT PROTECTION POLICY AND PROCEDURES

When the local multi-agency Adult Protection policy and procedures were developed and implemented in Norfolk, guidance was developed for practitioners concerning matters of confidentiality, the recording of information and the monitoring systems for capturing information concerning situations of abuse. The guidance was written to accompany the procedures, in order to assist in the ease of use in everyday practice. Introduction to the guidance as well as the procedures therefore also formed part of training sessions on adult protection for practitioners. As the policy and procedures applied to all social care settings, practitioners from all of those settings also participated in the training sessions.

Assessment is considered fundamental to the process of protection planning (Department of Health, 2000a; Penhale et al., 2000). Where allegations are received, from whatever source, which suggest that an adult is at risk of, or has suffered, abuse or neglect, enquiries must be made to ascertain the risk, or the potential risk, to the person, and the actions, if any, to be taken to protect and promote their welfare. Initially, as much information as possible should be gathered from the referrer.

INFORMATION GATHERING AND ASSESSMENT

As we saw in Chapter 5 on assessment, in deciding whether to take action to safeguard an adult at risk, careful gathering and assessment of information needs to take place. This is in order to evaluate whether the person is suffering harm or exploitation, and whether intervention is in the best interests of the person and/or in the public interest.

The following factors should be considered:

- the risk to the individual and their capacity to make their own decisions
- the nature and extent of the abuse or neglect; severity of abuse
- the length of time it has been occurring
- the impact on the individual(s)
- the risk of repeated or increasingly serious acts involving this individual or other adults at risk of abuse or neglect.

Whenever abuse or neglect of an adult is alleged or suspected, it is important to consider whether any other adults could be at risk of abuse or neglect. The need for a large-scale assessment and investigation is evident where it is suspected that a number of adults have been abused or neglected:

• in the same setting
• by the same perpetrator
• by a group of perpetrators

In these circumstances it is likely that a number of different agencies will need to be involved and work in a co-ordinated way. The process will be likely to consist of a number of individual assessments and investigations, some of which may need to be jointly undertaken across agencies.

Thus the full assessment occurs after the initial investigation and requires joint decision-making and planning, setting out the necessary steps to ensure future safety. It will also specify any treatment, therapies and services to be made available and future support plans and risk management strategies. However, we can also visualise assessment involving three interlocking processes: social assessment, risk assessment and decision-making (see Figure 6.1).

Decision-making is central to effective work with people in need of protection. This involves making plans. Social care agencies have procedures in place that ensure that plans are drawn up. When plans are undertaken together with service users it helps to ensure accountability and openness. It also provides a valuable way of changing and developing plans in ways that will meet identified needs. Used in an unthinking manner

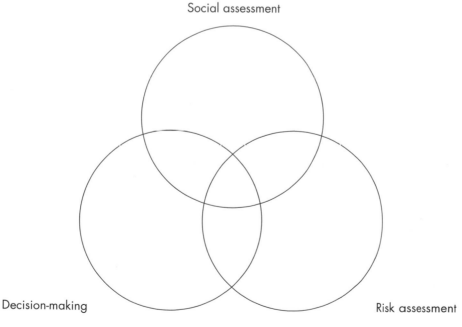

FIGURE 6.1 Three interlocking processes of assessment

solely to fulfil the obligations of the agency, a care plan is likely to reflect the wants, wishes and views of the individual practitioner rather than the service user and may therefore further victimise the service user. As with all forms of social care practice, developing a care plan is only as good as the processes involved in its formation and the value base of the practitioners and agency developing the plan.

Whilst agencies will have developed plans to reflect their work, it must be remembered that each plan is unique to the people and situations involved. Having said this, a safety or protection plan is likely to include the following:

- details of the services and interventions to be provided
- details of who will be involved in service delivery and provision
- a named co-ordinator
- other contact points
- measures and monitoring criteria
- a complaints and review procedure
- a review date.

Case studies follow, giving examples of financial exploitation and of rights, values and a case of neglect.

CASE STUDY 6.3:   AGNES

Agnes Martin was admitted to a residential home after a period in hospital, as she was unable to return to live alone at home. She received regular visits from several members of her family. One day following a visit a member of care staff found Agnes in her room, clearly very upset. Agnes said that she had talked to one of her daughters about her personal allowance from the Benefits Agency, as she had not received this. Her daughter, Joan, had said that she was receiving the money on behalf of Agnes and was saving this for her. When Agnes had asked where the money was, Joan had changed her story several times but had said that she would bring some of the money next time she visited. Agnes thought that Joan did not have any intention of bringing the money and that she had probably spent it as her family were experiencing financial problems. When Joan failed to bring the money at her next visit, Agnes talked with her key worker about the situation and they devised a plan to try and obtain the money from Joan and to safeguard her personal allowance in future. This protection plan was recorded and kept with Agnes's care plan and records. As Agnes wished to avoid any intervention by the police, the matter was dealt with by the care staff in the home following liaison with the local inspection and registration office (CSCI) and the local district social services office.

___

CASE STUDY 6.4: JO

___

Jo Dickson, a hospital social worker, received a referral from a ward concerning an eighty-seven-year-old man, Harry Davies. He had been admitted to the ward from a care home where he had lived for the last eighteen months. On admission he was immobile and was found to be malnourished, dehydrated and with very severe bedsores. His condition was so bad that photographs of his physical state had been taken, with the permission of his family. Harry's daughter had asked to see a social worker and wished to complain about her father's treatment in the home. In the last few months, following a change of ownership and management, her father had been moved to a room on the second floor with no lift access and had been unable to leave his room without physical assistance, as he was wheelchair-bound. Although Harry and the family had voiced their concerns about this matter and complained to the home, no action had been taken. Gradually it had reached a point where Harry seemed to have been almost forgotten by the care staff; meals were served erratically and it appeared that he sometimes went for at least half a day without liquid or getting out of bed. His physical condition had deteriorated in recent weeks, leading to his hospital admission. The family wished to know whom to complain to about the home and were given advice and information about the local registration and inspection unit (now CSCI). They also wished to make arrangements for Harry to move to another home and were given advice about this too. The Registration unit investigated the situation, with supporting evidence from the hospital staff, and the owners of the home were forced to make some major changes to the home in order to maintain their registration. One senior member of staff was sacked by the home and was later disciplined by the NMC (the professional body for Nursing and Midwifery). Unfortunately Harry died in hospital; ongoing social work support was given to the family for a period following this situation.

WORKING TOGETHER IN ADULT PROTECTION

It has been the policy of a number of UK governments for many years now that there should be increasing inter-agency collaboration between health and social services, and this has been well reported elsewhere (Balloch and Taylor, 2001; Hudson and Hardy, 2002; Clarke and Glendinning, 2003; Quinney, 2006). This policy of moving towards increased partnership working and integrated forms of service delivery is viewed as having the following types of advantages: the provision of best-quality and most effective care for those people who require multiple services, reducing duplication or overlap between services and preventing people from falling through gaps in service provision (Edwards and Miller, 2003). More recently, the drive towards greater partnership working has begun to move beyond the level of encouragement or even exhortation by government within policies, as previously found (Loxley, 1997), to being enshrined in law, for example through the Community Care Act, 2003, the Health and Social Care Act, 2001, and the Police Reform Act, 2002.

Further to this the Local Government White Paper, 2006, has proposed a range of measures in order to improve partnership working between local authorities and health services. This is in order to assist in securing the development of integrated care services across the social care sector and throughout the country. A new duty to co-operate for local authorities and primary care trusts within the new statutory health and well-being partnerships will be introduced. The White Paper suggests that this statutory duty to co-operate will lead to the achievement of shared outcomes, joint commissioning of services and also eventually, single budgets in localities. In addition to these developments we have already also seen the legal duty for safeguarding children moved to a number of key organisations rather than resting solely with social services through the introduction of the Children Act, 2004 (Goldthorpe, 2004). At present, however, as we will see below, at a strategic level this does not appear to have extended to the area of adult protection.

In 1998, the government introduced a framework for its agenda to modernise social care services (Department of Health, 1998b). Amongst these initiatives, one of the key areas identified as in need of modernisation related to the need to improve systems of protection for users of social care services, in particular those people who might be identified as vulnerable. The major intention of this part of the agenda was to ensure that vulnerable people receiving social care services could be certain that the care received was supplied in ways that were both competent and safe. This should be the case no matter where the service is delivered, in a person's own home or in a care setting. There was also a concern to ensure that vulnerable adults were protected from other forms of abuse (that is not relating to the provision of care services).

When the guidance document *No Secrets* was introduced in England in 2000 (a similar document, *In Safe Hands*, was issued in Wales during the same year), there was a very clear emphasis on the need for a number of different agencies to work together in order to produce effective solutions to situations of adult abuse or to decrease the risk of abuse of individuals who might be considered to be vulnerable (Department of Health, 2000a; National Assembly for Wales, 2000). Indeed the documents were signed by two ministers of Health (for Health and Social Services respectively) and the Home Office minister in order to underline the importance of having a joined-up approach to adult protection. It also highlighted the need for multi-agency working in this area.

As we have seen in Chapter 3 on the law and Chapter 4 on regulation, a large number of changes have been introduced in the course of the last few years, which have an impact on adult protection. Developments relating to criminal justice such as *Action for Justice* initiatives (Home Office, 2001), and those relating to vulnerable victims within *Achieving Best Evidence* (Home Office, 2003) as well as within community safety and domestic violence, have had an impact on adult protection practices. Changes in legislation, for example the Sexual Offences Bill, and other developments, such as the implementation of the Care Standards Act, 2000, the establishment of the Criminal Records Bureau, the development of the Commission for Social Care Inspection (soon to join with the Commission for Healthcare Audit and Inspection), the General Social Care Council, the Commission for Health Improvement and the National Patient Safety Agency also need to be examined from an adult protection perspective. The development of the Single Assessment Process, which has developed as part of the National Service Framework for Older People, is also relevant here as the framework emphasises the need for clear processes of inter-agency information exchange and in addition there are assessment items concerning protection and safety included within the process. Thus there are a number of different systems relating to adult protection that need to be linked in with such developments. All of the above organisations impact on the work of those agencies involved in adult protection, albeit to differing degrees. Indeed, most, if not all, agencies that deal with adult service users are involved to some extent in the prevention, investigation and management of concerns around adult protection and vulnerable adults. It is therefore important to consider the need for multi agency work in this area a little further.

Although we have mentioned national-level organisations, which may need to link with adult protection processes, it is perhaps at local level that the need for joint working becomes most apparent. Multi-agency and multidisciplinary work with vulnerable adults has existed for a number of years now as we will see in chapters concerning learning disability and mental health, where there are now often integrated teams undertaking such work. It may therefore appear fairly obvious that joint working should also exist within adult protection, but this does not yet seem to be a routine occurrence throughout the country. No Secrets provided a mandate for local authority Social Services Departments (as they were then called) to assume the lead role for the co-ordination of responses to adult protection concerns and referrals in each area. Although this is a statutory mandate for social services (under section 7 of the Local Authority and Social Services Act, 1970), which means that it is a requirement for them to undertake this role, unfortunately it is not a statutory requirement for the other agencies at local level to be involved, so the guidance in No Secrets remains guidance, with some degree of permissiveness for those other agencies and it would seem some degree of choice concerning the extent of involvement in multi-agency working.

In most areas, it would appear that, in line with the guidance document, local Adult Protection Committees (APCs) have been set up in recent years (although they may not all be known as Adult Protection Committees, but may have other names such as Multi-agency Management Committee or Safeguarding Board). These are indicative of the collaborative arrangements that have been established between organisations involved in adult protection. Indeed a recent survey of all authorities in England and Wales, undertaken by Penhale and colleagues, found that 96 per cent of authorities had committees in place by 2004–5 (Perkins et al., 2007). A further 2 per cent of authorities reported that they had plans to establish a committee within the next six months and only a very small number, 1 per cent, stated that they had no plans to set up a committee, but gave no reason for this. This survey had an 84 per cent response rate, including 100 per cent from Welsh authorities, and therefore the information obtained can be viewed as reasonably representative of the situation in the country as a whole.

However, the survey also found that the number of organisations represented on these committees varied a great deal. The number of different agencies on APCs ranged from three to sixteen with an average of nine different agencies represented on the committee. Representatives from Social Services or from Councils with Social Services Responsibilities (CSSRs) were present on each committee, which is perhaps not surprising since Social Services have the lead responsibility for co-ordinating responses and the guidance document was clear that one effective way of achieving co-ordinated work was to have some form of management committee. Therefore in most authorities it has been Social Services that have set up these committees. From the survey responses, it is clear that the vast majority of committees also included representatives from health (97 per cent) and the police (93 per cent) at local level. Just over three-quarters of APCs (76 per cent) had representatives from inspection and regulatory bodies (i.e. CSCI or CSIW, which is the equivalent organisation in Wales) and a slightly lower proportion (70 per cent) had representatives from Primary Care Trusts (PCTs) on committees. Owing to the somewhat amorphous nature of health organisations, it was decided to separate out PCT and Mental Health Trust representation on committees. However, health representation could also include Strategic Health Authority and/or Acute Trust representation as well as PCT or Mental Health Trusts, and it is these bodies that appear to make up the bulk of health representation on committees as Mental Health Trust representation was reported by only 37 per cent of respondents.

Charitable and voluntary organisations were found to be present on 65 per cent of committees. However, fewer than a third of APCs (30 per cent) had some form of carer or service-user representation, and fewer than 10 per cent of APCs (9 per cent) had representation from special interest groups (e.g. black minority ethnic or other specific community groups). Only 5 per cent of committees had separate representation from domestic violence organisations.

In addition to the broad range of organisations represented on committees reported in the survey, there was also a wide variation in relation to the frequency of APC meetings. Most APCs met on a quarterly basis (56 per cent) whilst just under a quarter of committees (22 per cent) met every two months. Six per cent of APCs met less than twice a year and 3 per cent met on a six-weekly basis. Only 1 per cent met monthly and only 2 per cent met on a four-monthly basis. The mean number of APC meetings held by committees per year was four.

Additionally, it must be noted that, although a committee may have a large number of potential attenders, it may well be that not all organisations are likely to attend every meeting or to have nominated deputies to attend if the principal person is not able to attend. From a further section of the survey, the most frequently mentioned barrier to multi-agency working in adult protection was the lack of commitment that some agencies showed towards working together in multi-agency groups, which was identified by over half of the respondents (58 per cent). It also appears that attendance at committee meetings by representatives from other organisations at the appropriate level can prove problematic at times. For example if the committee is trying to operate at a strategic level and take decisions about organisational commitment, such as available resources, then clearly attendance by senior level staff is likely to be necessary. Yet in some authorities which participated in the study, it is apparent that relatively junior staff attend meetings, who are not really able to participate in strategic-level discussions or to take decisions. As this quote demonstrates:

> Acute trusts have attended committee meetings, but [they] have sent junior staff and it has been a struggle to get each trust to take it seriously and to have procedures for their staff.
>
> (LA 50)

A number of the survey respondents in the section of the survey which invited free text responses in relation to the barriers experienced in working together spoke of the reluctance shown by some agencies to work together or the uncertainty that they seemed to experience in relation to disclosing information. As one respondent noted:

[The] Department of Works and Pensions [are] still rigid to their data protection policy despite the huge rise in financial abuse coming to light.

(LA 38)

Another respondent stated: 'Probably the biggest barrier to multi-agency working is where there is concern about information sharing . . . trust between agencies is a must' (LA 110).

Yet the need for the sharing of information across different organisations has been well established in recent years (Richardson and Asthana, 2005) and in many areas there are now both statutory provisions and practice frameworks that relate to information sharing and the disclosure of service users' personal information across agencies. So for example, agencies are required to take necessary measures to safeguard personal information, such as agreeing to implement the Caldicott standard (see below), and to reach agreement about information sharing protocols to be used at local level. These protocols must take account of and adhere to the requirements of legislation such as the Data Protection Act, 1998, the Freedom of Information Act, 2000, and the Human Rights Act, 1998, as well as guidance from the Department for Constitutional Affairs (2003).

In the late 1990s, the growing number of people in the healthcare team and the increasing use of electronic data storage and retrieval led to concerns about the safety and confidentiality of patient information. An inquiry to consider these issues was chaired by Dame Fiona Caldicott. The subsequent report recommended that all NHS trusts and Health Authorities should appoint a Caldicott Guardian to ensure that high standards of protection for confidential clinical information were regularly and objectively assessed and maintained. This is an important element of good clinical governance (Department of Health, 1999b). The concept has since been implemented within social care environments (Department of Health, 2002b).

In addition, several of the respondents cited practical difficulties that affected agencies in maintaining continuity (for example regularly attending meetings) or simply said that some agencies lacked commitment. One respondent observed that different policy priorities could impact on the level of engagement of an organisation: 'It is not given priority in the NHS as it does not attract any star ratings' (LA 50).

An overlapping concern, and the second principal barrier, was the degree of variation amongst participating agencies in the priority that was given to adult protection work, which was cited by just under half of respondents (43 per cent). This variation in prioritising adult protection was said to affect the degree of shared ownership of adult protection work and the degree of shared responsibility that it was possible to achieve. As one respondent stated: 'Currently adult protection committee meetings are not well attended, suggesting a lack of commitment when other priorities are at stake' (LA 56). It would appear that, because there is not a statutory requirement for all relevant organisations to be involved in adult protection work, adult protection work takes a back seat at times when other priorities occur. In a later qualitative phase of the study undertaken by Penhale et al., information was provided in a number of different areas across England and Wales that strongly indicated that at times both police and health organisations refused or were unable to take part in or continue to be involved in adult protection investigations as other, higher priorities had arisen for those organisations (Penhale et al., 2007).

However, although these results may give a somewhat negative view about inter-agency work in this area, it must be noted that a small proportion of respondents (9 per cent) stated that there were no barriers at all to multi-agency working and that in general, as we shall see below, multi-agency work in adult protection was viewed very positively by the majority of survey respondents.

In relation to a question about the strengths of working together within adult protection, the strength most frequently identified by respondents was the area of shared expertise (81 per cent). This included sharing knowledge or information with other adult protection committee members, as well as sharing resources and training. As one respondent stated:

> [It] vastly improves capacity to weigh risks and address them effectively. Vastly increases options available to protect and support . . . if someone chooses to remain at risk. Sharing at a strategic level widens understanding of policy and implementation options.
>
> (LA 13)

In response to an open question, some respondents indicated that multi-agency working provided the opportunity to widen views and understanding through taking account of other agencies' perceptions and considered that this also helped to break down barriers between agencies. As this respondent indicated:

> Through the [vulnerable adults] policy we have broken down barriers between agencies, particularly social services, the police and health and shared important information on a need to know basis which has significantly enhanced [the] working relationship and resulted in fuller, more co-operative investigations and better outcomes.
>
> (LA 38)

Just under three-quarters (72 per cent) of survey respondents reported that the second major strength of multi-agency working within committees was the development of a more effective approach to adult protection. Such an approach was said to include improvements in operational capacity and in decision-making, as well as establishing a more proactive approach towards adult protection within organisations. A third strength was considered to be the sense of shared responsibility that was produced by multi-agency working, and this was cited by over two-thirds (69 per cent) of respondents. Multi-agency working was seen as supplying a good way to reach consensus; it sped up decision-making, reduced work duplication and helped to create structures in which agencies could demonstrate a tangible commitment to adult protection. The fourth strength was a shared view from over half of respondents (56 per cent) that working together provided an approach towards adult protection that was strategically effective. Those respondents who cited this strength reported that multi-agency working was an essential approach, it was more consistent and systematic than single-agency working and it also provided important opportunities for future planning and development of adult protection processes and systems within local areas.

The survey indicated that a partnership approach was seen as beneficial to help protect vulnerable people. The reported benefits included:

- information sharing
- sharing of skills and expertise

- the fostering of shared ownership and responsibility in relation to adult protection amongst agencies, particularly in the areas of developing joint procedures and strategies.

However, respondents also identified barriers and disadvantages to working together. The main barriers and disadvantages that were reported were:

- agencies not being fully committed to multi agency working
- agencies not providing the resources required (either financial or human resources)
- lack of clarity with regard to the roles and responsibilities of each agency
- lack of information sharing protocols
- different priorities of agencies
- delays in decision-making at both strategic and operational levels because of the number of agencies involved.

Also of concern were:

- the lack of adequate resources for adult protection work
- the lack of statutory legislation to protect vulnerable adults
- the attitudes of some agencies that the guidance document was a 'may do' rather than a 'must do'.

In general terms, respondents viewed multi-agency working very positively. As one respondent stated: 'I really don't know what to say, I just can't imagine trying to do this any other way. In every single adult protection case we always need the skills, [and] experience [of] . . . more than one agency' (LA 77).

Many respondents echoed the sentiments behind this view in both the survey phase and the subsequent interview phase that took place in twenty-six different local authorities across England and Wales. It appeared that by far the majority of participants in the wider study were committed to the concept of inter-agency working in adult protection but that in practice achievement of this was not necessarily straightforward, owing largely it would seem to structural constraints. Partnership working within adult protection was viewed as something of an 'ideal state' to be strived for, as it was acknowledged that the attainment of effective co-ordinated and jointly planned services was difficult to achieve. This would also seem to be the case in sectors other than the area of adult protection (Fletcher, 2006). That co-ordination of both public sector and voluntary endeavours to benefit individuals who are in need of assistance or protection owing to some form of social vulnerability might be an appropriate approach to take did not appear to be in question within the study, particularly at the strategic level at which most committees operated.

There are various changes that appear likely to occur within the world of adult social care in coming years; indeed it sometimes seems that some sort of change is pretty much inevitable at any point in time! However, following the reorganisation of social services since the implementation of the Children Act, 2004, with the separation of services for children from adult services, and the suggestion that adult social care should be mixed with the wider agenda for public health and well-being (Cozens, 2006) it appears rather more difficult to define what adult social care practitioners are responsible for and who their service users are. This is important, as it is also apparent that the social care needs of adults cover a wide range and are very diverse. Adult social care practitioners and service providers therefore need to be particularly flexible in order to be able to respond to needs no matter when and how they arise. This is likely to be the case also within matters relating to safeguarding and adult protection. It also seems that given the well-being agenda there are likely to be demands for increasing inter-departmental working within councils, for example with leisure, transport and housing departments, and that there will also be a need to develop wide-ranging partnerships with external organisations in order to ensure that there is sufficient focus on social inclusion for those adults who are vulnerable or otherwise marginalised. Adult Protection Committees (or Safeguarding Boards) may be well placed to consider some of these issues in future, especially when these matters of social exclusion relate centrally to issues of needs for safety and protection. The need for such committees to increase levels of representation from the voluntary and independent sectors is therefore likely to be more apparent in future, and the imperative for partnership working (at strategic levels) and inter-agency working (at operational levels) will also be increasingly necessary within adult protection.

SUMMARY

Working with abuse in care settings is a complex matter. We have seen that there are a number of different ways in which practitioners may become involved and intervene in situations of poor practice or abuse. The suggestions made are not the only types of interventions, however, and practitioners need to be alert to the range of possibilities when facing such situations. It is also necessary to be aware of other possible sources of support and information, such as those provided by such organisations as Counsel & Care and Action on Elder Abuse. Both of these have produced information on abuse in care settings (Counsel & Care, 1995; Action on Elder Abuse, 2002) and provide useful sources of advice for concerned individuals. The organisation Public Concern at Work also provides advice concerning 'whistle-blowing' and in recent years has received an increasing number of calls from social care practitioners who wish to discuss concerns about abusive situations that they are coming across and where they are uncertain about what to do. Working together between the different relevant organisations involved is likely to become increasingly important in future within adult protection.

KEY READING

Clarke, J. and Glendinning, C. (2003) Partnerships and the remaking of welfare governance. In C. Glendinning, M. Powell and K. Rummery (eds) *Partnerships, New Labour and the Governance of Welfare*, Bristol: Policy Press.

Cozens, A. (2006) Use your imagination, *Community Care*, 19–25 October, 38–40.

Parker, J. (2007b) Social work, disadvantage by association and anti-oppressive practice. In P. Burke and J. Parker (eds) *Social Work and Disadvantage: Addressing the Roots of Stigma through Association*, London: Jessica Kingsley.

Penhale, B. and Parker, J. with Kingston, P. (2000) *Elder Abuse*, Birmingham: Venture Press.

CHAPTER 7

MENTAL HEALTH DIFFICULTIES

OBJECTIVES

By the end of this chapter you should:

- be able to describe social policy issues concerning people with difficulties relating to mental health and protection

- be able to detail how abuse may be experienced by people with mental health difficulties

- be able to consider the social and family perspectives in which abuse and protection are experienced

- be able to suggest a number of ways of working with people with mental health difficulties where there are issues relating to abuse and protection.

INTRODUCTION

A number of adults, but by no means all, have difficulties relating to their mental health which can lead to vulnerability and a need for protection. However, a number of individuals may at times have needs concerning their own safety (by their own actions or lack of actions) or the safety of others. The diversity of needs of individuals with mental health difficulties can be problematic for social care practitioners and policy-makers, given the need to consider each individual and also needs relating to public safety. This may present additional problems when there is a need to consider services for people with mental health difficulties, as we shall see later in the chapter, especially if there are issues relating to safety involved. This chapter first examines what mental health difficulties are, including some of the issues relating to definitions. It then explores current services for adults with mental health difficulties and this is followed by a consideration of risk, vulnerability, protection and abuse of adults with mental health difficulties and the ways in which practitioners respond to such issues. We will also look at the needs of informal carers (family members and friends) and the needs of adults who experience problems connected to mental health, especially where there are situations of abuse. As part of this exploration, we will also need to look at some of the ethical issues relating to autonomy, capacity and the right to take risks. However, we start with a case study.

CASE STUDY 7.1:   BRENDA

Brenda Smithson was in her late fifties when she was referred to the Social Services Department for assessment owing to a mental health problem. The referral came from her GP, who provided the following information. Brenda was an only child who had always lived with her parents and never left home. She had worked as an insurance clerk from the time she left school at sixteen until her late forties. At that time she stopped work in order to help her mother care for her father who was very ill and who died after several years of care from mother and daughter. Brenda had not been able to find work at this point and in any case soon had to look after her mother, who developed a heart condition and needed a lot of care and assistance. After six years of care, her mother had died, leaving Brenda on her own in the family home. Brenda had not managed the death of her father very well, as she was concerned at the time with making sure that her mother was all right, so the death of her mother after an intensive period of care was like a double loss to Brenda. In addition she had never been completely on her own before and had not had the responsibility of managing a house as well as herself and it soon became apparent that this was too much for her. Described as anxious from when she was a child, Brenda had always been a bit 'nervy' and could get very upset over very small matters. Her anxiety on losing her mother and being alone had increased dramatically and she was no longer able to cope. In fact, in order to try and cope, she had developed a number of obsessive-compulsive behaviours, such as continual hand-washing and checking routines, but these appeared to be escalating so that Brenda was not always able to leave the house, even for essential supplies.

The social worker who visited found that Brenda was indeed very anxious and acting in compulsive ways and that she had not left the house for several weeks as she did not feel it was safe to do so (something bad might happen to her or to the house whilst she was out). Although she was initially not very keen, Brenda accepted help from a home carer visiting regularly to do shopping, help with cleaning and also to reassure Brenda about her coping. Regular visits from a Community Psychiatric Nurse (CPN) were also arranged as well as social work visits to monitor the situation as Brenda refused to take any medication for her condition or to go to a day centre or hospital. She was worried that if she went to the local psychiatric hospital she would be kept there against her will, so it was safer for her to refuse to go and to insist that people visit her at home.

This case study is an individual account of someone developing a neurotic disorder over a period of time; indeed, we can see that in all likelihood Brenda's psychological health had been fragile since childhood. Her vulnerability, which also developed, was very much related to her own actions or lack of actions, rather than occurring from external people or events, but this still placed her at risk of harm, albeit from herself. However, her views about the psychiatric hospital are very common as people still equate psychiatric hospitals or asylums with people being locked up and unable to leave the institution, of being kept there against their will. Indeed, as many former work-houses became local psychiatric hospitals, community views of such places were already tainted from their very beginnings as asylums, as workhouses were places where individuals in need of either correction (for example unmarried mothers) or care (for example paupers with health conditions) were admitted and often kept living there for many years.

However, policies concerning care in the community were partly developed as a result of reactions to concern about the institutionalisation of individuals in long-stay hospitals. Although the majority of people living in long-stay hospitals and affected by such policies were adults with learning disabilities, the move towards people being cared for wherever possible in community settings, described in Chapter 2, relates also to adults with mental health difficulties. And as we shall see in Chapter 8, there were a number of reasons for the development of the framework for care in the community, leading to the closure of many large hospitals, institutions both for people with a learning disability and for people with mental health problems. Before we go further with this exploration, a discussion of definitions and terms appears to be in order.

WHAT IS MENTAL HEALTH AND MENTAL ILL-HEALTH?

Mental health is described by the World Health Organisation (WHO) in the following way:

> a state of well-being in which the individual realises his or her abilities, can cope with the normal stresses of life, can work productively and fruitfully, and is able to make a contribution to his or her community.
>
> Mental ill health includes mental health problems and strain, impaired functioning associated with distress, symptoms and diagnosable mental health disorders, such as schizophrenia and depression.
>
> The mental condition of people is determined by a multiplicity of factors including biological, individual, family and social economic and environmental.
>
> (WHO, 2001)

The case study at the beginning of this chapter appears to fit within this general description, as Brenda's mental health was adversely affected by her reactions to a combination of different factors.

It would appear that, at some time in their lives, around one in every six people in the UK will experience mental health difficulties that are serious enough for them to seek help from a professional (Social Trends, 2002). Generally, the first approach that people make is to their GP, or family doctor, but often the doctor will then refer individuals on to specialist psychiatric services or other agencies that provide mental health services. Such services include social work agencies as well as other health and social care agencies that are working together to provide services for those service users in need of them.

However, as we will also see in the next chapter, the use of specific terms and language itself can be undermining and oppressive towards people and in some instances may be considered as constituting psychological abuse. This needs to be borne in mind when we are discussing people with mental health difficulties, as some of the terms and language used have resulted in much stigma for those individuals. Although the terms used to describe people with mental health problems have changed considerably over time, so that for example people are not routinely referred to officially as 'lunatics' any longer, some of the language used is still problematic. Indeed, in the 1970s and 1980s, even the term 'mental illness' was questioned by those who considered that what was then described as madness was a problem caused by society and sometimes family processes (see for example the works of Laing and Esterson (1970) and Szasz (1972) in relation to this area) and this type of view has also resurfaced more recently within discussions on the social model of disability, including perspectives from mental health organisations (Sayce, 2003), although without the more distressing and unwarranted associations with family processes.

In relation to use of terms, it is important to consider non-professional perspectives and to look at the views that the general public have. Most information that the public obtain is derived from the media. Unfortunately, there have not been many studies that examine how ordinary people perceive and conceptualise mental health. One of the few studies that did look at this area discovered that people appear to view mental health and mental illness as part of the same broad continuum and also that, for many people, these terms seem to have negative connotations (Golightley, 2006).

ACTIVITY 7.1

Think about some of the coverage of mental illness you have seen in the media (television and films or videos as well as newspapers). Write down some of the most common words that you remember coming across. What terms are commonly used to describe mental disorder? Does this vary from less to more serious types of media?

You may have written down words like 'loony' or 'headcase' or 'nutter' which are all quite commonly used and which also generally have negative connotations both for the people using them and also for those to whom they are applied. Certain behaviours can become associated with particular labels and may then lead to what is known as a 'self-fulfilling prophecy'. This means that the behaviour is more likely to occur because of the term used and the expectation that this type of behaviour will result. What do you think about this? Is calling someone by one of these terms not detrimental and simply just fun, or might it result in some harm or offence to the person?

In addition to the broad description used by the WHO, however, we also need to consider that there are several different terms that may be used to describe the same thing. You may hear terms such as mental illness, mental distress, mental health problems and mental health difficulties used by professionals and most of these refer to more or less the same thing. A more global term would be mental disorder, which broadly covers any major departure from 'normal health' and includes a number of different illnesses and diseases. This includes serious conditions such as schizophrenia, or manic depression. But it also implies that the person had a normal state at some point in their lives, so it suggests that the disorder may well be of a temporary nature and that the person will be able to regain normality in future. It also implies that work can be undertaken with the person in order to help them regain that state. Mental health is a term that is difficult to be definitive about, however, as it is about more than just an absence of ill-health or illness. Probably the closest we can get to an ideal definition is about the ability to achieve the potential we have as human beings. Thus individuals can have mental health problems or difficulties that are, in effect, problems of everyday life and which need to be dealt with. Unfortunately this is easier for some people than for others, who may need assistance in order to cope and deal with such situations satisfactorily.

DIFFERENT MODELS OF MENTAL HEALTH AND ILLNESS

There are a number of different perspectives or models that are current within this area and it is necessary for you to have an understanding about the different models in use. This will mean that you can evaluate the different models used, and if you are working in this area you may also be able to locate your own practice within a relevant model. Essentially there are two main models that are used. These are:

- the medical model, which is generally held by medical (and some health) practitioners and is basically concerned with disease and biomedical approaches, and
- the social model, which is usually held by practitioners such as social workers and is inclined to look at social factors of causation and also considers labelling as a contributory factor.

However, since the implementation of community care in the mid-1990s (1993 onwards), an increasing number of health centres have mental health social workers attached to or working in them. This usually means that these workers will be out in the community, undertaking direct work with service users with mental health difficulties and often working together with mental health professionals with different (non-social-work) backgrounds. These social workers may also spend some of their time working in or at least visiting service users in local psychiatric hospitals, so it is useful that all social workers have some knowledge and understanding about the medical model. And although we have separated out the models, it is also important to state here that the medical model is the one which consistently continues to be dominant and so other views about mental health need to take this into account. It is to this model that we turn first.

The medical model

This is the model that is generally adopted by doctors (GPs) and psychiatrists and is also known as a disease model. This model accepts the claim made by clinical scientists that physical or organic causes will be found for all forms of mental disorder. The model has developed over the last 150 years or so since the time when doctors really began to treat and manage individuals with disorders of mental health. Prior to this time, when the state took control of the situation and doctors began to treat 'illness', people were generally seen within their communities as fools or eccentrics or as possessed by the devil (Scull, 1979).

Doctors within mental health settings are usually principally involved in the diagnosis of the disorder. Generally speaking, if the individual's behaviour gives rise to major concerns about the person's own safety or the safety of others, or is likely to need specialist services and maybe treatment such as medication in order to resolve or at least control it, then the person's GP will be likely to refer them to a psychiatrist for a specialist assessment and subsequent diagnosis of the condition. The diagnosis is usually made after quite lengthy contact between the doctor and the individual, perhaps lasting weeks or even months. The medical assessment, which contributes to the diagnosis, will include such aspects as any past history of mental health difficulties, the individual's view of the problem, other health conditions and family history of any disorders. One of the things that the doctor (or psychiatrist) will attempt to do is to decide whether there are particular signs and symptoms that the individual shows. This will assist in determining whether the person has mild or occasional difficulties or has more major and severe problems. One way of thinking about a diagnosis is as a sort of abbreviated description of what the psychiatrist decides or believes is the person's problem.

In order to try and ensure that the assessment processes used are not all different, doctors today commonly use specific tools for psychiatric assessment, often consisting of particular interview schedules. These have been standardised so that they are understood to be reliable and to give valid results. Such tools help in the detection of particular symptoms, which then provide indications for the doctor as to the diagnosis for that condition. Examples of such inventories are the Present State Examination (PSE) or the Beck Depression Inventory. The diagnosis should then lead to ongoing care and treatment (as necessary) and the involvement of other professionals such as social workers and community psychiatric nurses; it may also lead to the involvement of other agencies such as housing departments, if necessary.

Classifications of mental disorders

The classification of disorders, representing groups or patterns of symptoms, is an important adjunct to diagnosis. If groups of symptoms fit into an established and recognised pattern, they can be classified as a particular condition, such as depression, and a diagnosis made. This will also provide some clues and suggestions about what treatment might be needed and the management of the condition for both the doctor and the individual. Generally in the UK there are two main manuals of classification used: the ICD-10 (International Classification of Diseases, volume 10, developed by the World Health Organisation in 1992) and the DSM-IV (the Diagnostic and Statistical Manual of Mental Disorders, developed by the American Psychiatric Association). It is useful to know of the existence of such manuals and the basis on which diagnoses are made, even although you will not be likely to use these in your practice. However, despite attempts to ensure that these tools are both reliable and valid, disputes have still happened at various points in the years since their development and we need to recognise that as with other forms of assessment, there is a reliance on the amount and nature of the information provided. Insufficient or poor-quality information given will be likely to lead to an unsatisfactory result in terms of either an assessment or a diagnosis, so it may be necessary to maximise the quality of the information provided or obtained if at all possible (see Pritchard, 2006).

The social model

As we have seen above, the medical model considers mental disorder as an example of illness caused by a disease process (perhaps due to a viral cause), genetics or some other biomedical problem. The social model considers social, environmental or ecological factors that may lead to a disorder developing. So whereas the medical model is primarily concerned with looking at individuals and their particular pathology, the social model explores social reasons for causation. This means that issues relating to discrimination, oppression, power and social exclusion need to be considered as they are part of the social framework affecting many people, not just single individuals (Tew, 2002). The social model is therefore in accord with social work values relating to the use of holistic approaches, and this appears to be a fundamental principle for mental health social work as much as for other areas of social work. And although the social model is nowhere near as powerful as the medical model within mental health, it is very much viewed as the underlying basis for social work and social care practice in this area of work. In addition, if we consider the social model of disability in slightly more general terms, we see suggestions that what should develop is an understanding based on the disabling features of the society and environment rather than resulting from any condition in and of itself; this could equally apply to mental health as to other forms of disability.

However, even with the social model as it relates to mental health, there are a number of different perspectives that exist. These include such areas as labelling theory, social causation and social constructivism. We will expand on just two of these areas.

Labelling theory describes a process in which primary deviance occurs, such as odd or unusual behaviour, which continues and is then interpreted as secondary deviance or mental disorder. So for example, initial deviant or strange behaviour, which causes some concern, may be explained by another person in terms of an everyday understandable occurrence; thus bizarre behaviour may be explained by a partner as the person's way of getting rid of stress or 'letting off steam'. This means that some symptoms may be missed by doctors as well as by partners, as behaviours that are outside the norm for that person are treated as what should be happening, not what is actually happening to them. Secondary deviance may then occur when a diagnosis is made and the person takes on a deviant role. Just as in primary deviance the behaviour is interpreted as normal for the person, in secondary deviance the behaviour comes to be seen as behaviour that is typical for a person who has a mental disorder. In his seminal work, *Asylums*, Goffman talks about such situations as this as the making of a psychiatric patient (1961), and, as we saw in Chapter 1, he also discussed the way that a hospital may become or act as a total institution.

ACTIVITY 7.2

Take a few moments to reconsider Goffman's views about total institutions as cited in Chapter 1. Then, thinking about hospital settings, in particular those relating to mental health and psychiatry, write down some of the aspects that link such places to the description of total institutions.

You may have written down such notions as rigid or fixed routines, locked doors, lack of choice for patients, people not being able to wear their own clothes or even to do what they want. Whilst most admission wards in hospitals would now say that they do provide choice for individuals, that they can wear their own clothes and choose what time they go to bed (within reason!), on some wards there may still be more rigid routines and locked doors on occasion, if not all the time. You may also find it helpful to arrange to visit a psychiatric hospital if you have never done so; your college or work place may help to arrange this for you or even for a small group of students.

Perspectives considering social causation try to assist in considering the inter-action between mental disorder and social disadvantage. In this sort of view, the medical diagnosis of the person's condition is generally accepted, but the social scientist is concerned to examine the effects that different types of social disadvantage and inequality may have on the person's condition, in this case their mental health. Within this type of viewpoint it is also possible to include other important variables such as class, ethnicity and gender and consider what effects these may have on the person's mental health and their overall situation.

An examination of the concentration of people who are diagnosed with schizophrenia in inner-city areas is an example of this view relating to social causation. It has been discovered that a combination of social and economic factors can have an impact on the course of this disorder (Kelly, 2005). It appears that people from lower socio-economic groups are younger when they first present with the illness and are more likely not to engage with services; both of these factors seem to indicate poorer outcomes of treatment and overall prognosis over time. However, although it would appear that the incidence of schizophrenia is higher in inner-city areas than in suburban areas, and that it is predominantly a disorder that affects people in lower social classes, there is not a direct causal relationship between these factors and the condition and there are a number of possible explanations of relevance here. Work by Eaton (1980) identified the 'downward social drift' of people with schizophrenia so that it seems that people with the disorder migrate (or drift) into cities where they perhaps stand out less and where services are more likely to be found. In addition, people from higher social classes may be unable to maintain their positions owing to the effects of the illness over time, which are often quite devastating, and drift into the lower social classes then occurs. On the other hand, it could be that living in poverty in cities is much more difficult for people to withstand than poverty in rural areas and this then leads to a rise in the number of incidences of the illness in city areas.

Within the social model framework it is also useful to spend a few moments considering mental health and offending behaviour. As long ago as the 1930s it was suggested that, within most societies, levels of need for mental health institutions would be likely to remain fairly constant (Penrose, 1939). Therefore in a society with a well resourced mental health care system, a person who acts in a very bizarre or challenging way will be likely to be admitted to hospital. If, however, such services do not exist to meet such need, individuals will be more likely to be dealt with by the criminal justice system as an alternative means of dealing with a person deemed to be in need of social control. This situation seems familiar with the experiences of community care policies from the 1990s onwards; for example, Gunn (2004) has highlighted that we have seen a steady reduction in the number of formal psychiatric beds over the past twenty years, but a continuing increase in the number of mentally ill offenders and an increase in the general prison population of prisoners with major mental health problems. It is likely that this situation has arisen because, although hospital provision for people with mental health problems has decreased, there are not sufficient resources and services to assist people in community settings so the need for treatment may not be met, leading to a deterioration in mental health conditions. And in a consideration of the overlap between mental health and criminal justice systems, Wolff (2005) presents a rather grim view of services which are fragmented, large numbers of prisoners with severe mental health problems and a concentration of people with the most complex needs in the most deprived areas of our cities.

Furthermore, in a government report on social exclusion, the barriers that prevent individuals with severe mental health problems from being considered as 'full citizens' are emphasised (ODPM, 2004). The following factors are included: social isolation, issues relating to stigma and discrimination and lack of access to housing, employment and training. Galtung and Tord (1971) coined the term 'structural violence' to describe a built-in feature of social systems relating to inequalities in power and life chances. More recently, Kelly has used the term to describe the impact on the life chances and health, including mental health, of particular communities of such interrelated factors as poverty, racism and stigma (Kelly, 2005). In addition, a history of offending behaviour can also be considered to be a significant barrier to inclusion and of course the effects of such factors are likely to be further increased and perhaps even reinforced by the presence of mental health problems.

We also need to spend a little time considering issues relating to ethnicity and mental health. In addition to the stigma and discrimination that people with mental health problems are likely to experience, these difficulties can be deepened if the person also comes from a black or minority ethnic community. Keating and Robertson (2004) have detailed the views of black service users of mental health services and established that people perceive that they are worthless on account of their ethnicity. And, as we saw in Chapter 3, if a black person is considered to have a mental disorder and to display challenging behaviour, they are much more likely to receive secondary care in hospital and also to be detained in hospital against their wishes (Nazroo, 1999). It also seems that there is an underrepresentation of treatment of such individuals within primary care settings in the community rather than in hospital settings.

If mental health services are to be really responsive to the needs of individuals with mental health problems, then such services must respond to the needs of the diversity of individuals that live in the UK. As long ago as the late 1980s there were moves towards developing services that were more patient-centred, but these did not really respond to the particular needs of individuals from ethnic communities, and subsequent developments at policy levels since have not fully addressed such difficulties (Department of Health, 1999a; 2003b).

The bio-psycho-social model

Although we have looked at both the medical model and the social models of mental health, most practitioners working in this area would now consider that the most likely cause of mental health problems for an individual is a complex interaction of a range of different factors and that these are likely to include biological, psychological and social elements. Such factors could include the following components:

- biological vulnerability factors that predispose the person; these include genetic factors, biological elements and family or personal histories of mental health difficulties
- social factors including social class, experiences of racism or other forms of discrimination and social exclusion as components that may exacerbate mental health difficulties
- psychological factors including adverse reactions to loss, problematic relationships, lack of support networks or dysfunctional networks that may trigger mental health difficulties.

It is apparent that not all factors are likely to exist for any one individual and these examples are to give some idea of the range of factors that might be implicated in the onset and continuation of mental disorder. Factors from the different domains are likely to interact with each other, however, and may then determine whether a person develops good or poor mental health, whether they have the coping strategies to deal successfully with such difficulties or the resilience or protective factors to ensure that such difficulties either do not develop or do not cause major disruption to the individual's ability to function with situations of everyday life.

Looking at the range of different factors that might be involved for individuals means that it is possible to consider these with people and to establish what might be done in order to help them to achieve a good or positive mental health status. It is also possible to see how different people may experience broadly similar circumstances and yet react differently. For example, although an individual may have a family history of mental health problems, they may have a supportive social network and a job which is productive and which they find satisfying. The interaction between the factors may mean that the person does not experience these as vulnerability factors but rather as protective against developing a mental disorder. Conversely, there could be a situation where, although there may be an absence of any history of established mental health difficulties, major relationship difficulties or social exclusion due to a problem of substance misuse and the stress linked to such factors as these could result in an increase in the individual's vulnerability to develop mental health problems. And of course, if the weighting of such factors is predominantly negative, it may be much more likely that the person develops poor self-esteem, low resilience to difficult or problem factors and ultimately an increased possibility of developing poor mental health.

ACTIVITY 7.3

Reread the case study at the beginning of this chapter and examine the factors relating to Brenda that interacted in relation to her mental health. Consider the different elements involved to see whether there were relevant factors involved from biological, social or psychological spheres that may have interacted to produce her mental health problems.

Although you do not have all the information that might assist you with this exercise, it is important to recognise that trying to analyse such situations is generally complex and that evidence to support your analysis of the individual and their situation may be partial and collected over a period of time, during ongoing assessments of an individual and their situation. Likewise, the evidence that is obtained may then lead you to consider whether this factor (whatever it may be) could make the person more vulnerable or less vulnerable to developing a mental health problem.

It is also important to acknowledge the role of stress here as an intervening variable. Just as we have said that different people are likely to experience events that are similar in different ways, stress may also play an important role in relation to this in determining whether a person develops a mental health problem or not (Cochrane, 1983). It is not just the experience itself but the impact that this has on you and how you perceive and understand the event that has occurred (what meaning you ascribe to the situation) which is important to consider. If a person is not able to deal effectively with stress and becomes overstressed by difficult circumstances, they may not have adequate or sufficient coping strategies to manage and reduce the stress and this may contribute to the development of a mental health problem. Although it is probably impossible to help a person to entirely get rid of negative events or even to reduce them to an absolute minimum, it is usually possible to assist them to improve their strategies to manage or cope with the situations that cause them severe stress and therefore also to reduce their reactions to stressful events. Approaches such as stress management and relaxation techniques can assist people who are clearly vulnerable to such factors as these, which may serve to reinforce or worsen existing difficulties in this area.

In terms of preventing mental ill health, it would seem that there are two broad approaches that are helpful (Newton, 1988). First, work can be undertaken with individuals in order to reduce their vulnerability factors: this would include social workers being placed in specific preventive projects such as community initiatives to reduce social disadvantage and work on assisting people to increase their self-esteem and reduce social exclusion. Alternatively, work may take place to assist individuals to react more positively to situations and to develop improved resilience to stressful situations, such as may be found in projects that are linked to mental health improvement or 'healthy lifestyles' that include a mental health component. In many ways both of these approaches involve politics (with a small 'p') as many of the social factors that can affect people adversely are such things as poverty, unemployment and social exclusion. Work undertaken in projects may, however, counter some of the social disadvantages that people experience, as well as improving and promoting positive mental health for individuals.

MENTAL HEALTH STRATEGY AND POLICY

In general terms in recent decades successive governments can be said to have tried to improve mental health care. As stated earlier in the chapter, reforms have been taking place for more than twenty years in terms of trying to improve conditions for those people who are receiving care in hospitals, and we have also seen the movements to decrease the number of long-stay institutions and to introduce increasing amounts of care and services within community settings. Prior to this, the majority of care was provided in psychiatric hospitals, many of which were based in former workhouse sites and found on the edge of towns and cities. Following the development and implementation of community care policies in the 1980s and 1990s, moves have been made to shift the principal axis of care to community settings and for people to remain living in the community, rather than be routinely shut away from the public gaze in hospitals. Since the Labour Party was elected to government in 1997, a large number of policy documents have been published and implemented and, as we will see later, successive attempts to reform the mental health legislation and to update the Mental Health Act, 1983.

Amongst the policy documents that have been introduced are *Modernising Mental Health Services* (Department of Health, 1998c) and *The National Health Plan* (Department of Health, 2000b). One of the major intentions of such policies is to shift service provisions so that they are really user-focused, whilst at the same time tackling the effects of social exclusion on individuals with mental health problems. The overall intention is that through a combination of different initiatives introduced by a number of policy changes, individuals will feel less excluded and will then have more sense of belonging to the communities they live in. Services would then be able to form new collaborations and partnerships between service providers and service users. Thus a number of initiatives have been introduced to meet the needs of particular groups of service users with mental health problems such as black and minority ethnic groups and women.

At the end of the 1990s the National Service Framework (NSF) was developed and introduced. This consists of a number of key target areas for improvements in the health of the nation. And central to our discussion here is the *National Service Framework for Menthal Health* (Department of Health, 1999a), which serves as a series of targets for services in a number of distinct areas. There are NSFs relating to older people, adults of working age and children and young people. Each of these contains a number of specific standards that services should attain. So for example, the NSF for adult mental health has seven standards (see Box 7.1).

BOX 7.1   NATIONAL SERVICE FRAMEWORK FOR MENTAL HEALTH STANDARDS

Standard 1 covers health promotion (connected to mental health) and aspects of social exclusion and discrimination that are related to mental health problems.

Standards 2 and 3 are concerned with primary care services, including 24-hour crisis provision for individuals with mental health problems.

Standards 4 and 5 emphasise the essential elements of effective services for adults in need and include discussion of the Care Programme Approach and the link between this and care management systems in social care.

Standard 6 covers the needs of individuals who provide care for people with mental health problems, that is informal or unpaid care givers. Social Services Departments have the lead responsibility in ensuring that the needs of carers are appropriately assessed and that they receive their own provision, including care plans, where necessary.

Standard 7 relates to initiatives to reduce the number of suicides.

Although these standards are specific to mental health, and in particular adult mental health, there is regular monitoring of progress towards the achievement of the standards and overall this progress is overseen by a 'Tsar' (or champion) for mental health. There are also links to other standards, largely relating to inspection, that have been developed by the Commission for Social Care Standards (which as the renamed Commission for Social Care Inspection is also linked to the Healthcare Commission and the Audit Commission, which are other arms of government which monitor and evaluate service provision, public services and so forth).

A further major policy initiative of relevance here was introduced during 2005 and 2006 (Department of Health, 2005a; 2006a). In 2005, a consultation document was published by the Department of Health and this was followed by a White Paper which appeared in 2006, which was based on the ideas contained in the consultative Green Paper. The resultant White Paper, *Our Health, Our Care, Our Say: A New Direction for Community Services*, is an important document that sets out a new direction for health and social care systems as they relate to adult services. It indicates a major change in the way that services should be provided to people, with service users placed more centrally than previously and arguably viewed as being at the heart of service provision. This means that services should be more individualised and tailored to individual needs, progressing the direction that was first signalled in the community care reforms of the 1990s. There are four principal goals set out in the White Paper. These are:

- prevention and early intervention: this will include higher levels of support to maintain and promote mental health and psychological or emotional well-being

- more choice and more voice, which aims to provide improved levels of 'real choice' for service users from an expanded range of services and also the provision of improved levels of information, to enable individuals to make informed choices about their care
- removing inequalities and improving access, principally concerned with individuals with needs relating to ethnicity or long-term disabilities
- improved and higher levels of support for individuals with long-term needs so that they can self-manage long-term conditions in community settings.

Clearly this agenda is wide-ranging and potentially far-reaching. It remains to be seen, of course, how these policy changes will be implemented in the coming years, but potentially there could be major changes for the provision of care to adult service users, whether they have mental health problems or long-term (physical) health conditions.

In general terms, in the last two decades legislative and policy reform for mental health has demonstrated some difficulty in distinguishing between control and regulation within both institutional and community settings as the dominant theme for the content of emerging legislation and policy within mental health services, as seen in the Mental Health Patients in the Community Act, 1995, and Mental Health Bill, 2006 (Department of Health, 1995; 2006b). This would appear to have resulted in an apparent over-emphasis on public protection from mentally ill people, rather than perceiving people with mental illness as possibly vulnerable to abuse and perhaps in need of protection and safety themselves.

THE NEEDS OF CARERS FOR PEOPLE WITH MENTAL HEALTH PROBLEMS

Care giving for an individual with complex needs, be this in relation to individuals with physical or mental health difficulties, can be a very difficult task. The nature of the tasks involved is such that the role may be physically very demanding, for example in the situation of a person with problems in relation to physical health or disability or with multiple conditions. Or it may be psychologically and emotionally demanding, which may perhaps be more likely for a care giver for a person with a long-term and quite possibly severe mental health problem (Lefley, 1987; 1996). Of course, this is not to say that there are not both physical and mental health components to different forms of care giving, but rather that one or other form may predominate at particular times and for particular conditions. So, for example, if a care giver has to get up at night to tend to someone with physical problems that mean that they need to be turned over in bed at night, this is likely to be both physically tiring and also emotionally wearing owing to lack of sleep and broken nights. If the person has a mental health problem that requires intensive (if not constant) supervision during the daytime, this may not be physically tiring in quite the same way, although there is likely to be a physical component to the care provided, but it will be likely to be extremely emotionally and psychologically exacting.

In addition family care givers are also likely to experience strong emotional reactions to the illness of the person they are caring for, as there are often elements of loss and grief involved in relation to the particular condition. Examples of these aspects include the loss of good health and possible premature death of the person, the loss of the 'normal healthy person' and of the previous relationship, as well as the effects of living with uncertainty in terms of prognosis and at times perhaps bizarre and unpredictable behaviours (perhaps of a person with a mental health condition). Of course if a person has always had the particular condition, rather than recently developing it, there may not be the same element of grieving the loss of the previously healthy person, but there may be a perceived loss of the normal person (who never was) or the lack of possibility of a relationship which is not based on care giving.

All of these factors may be stressful for the principal care giver and for other family members to deal with and may also have an effect on the care giver's own health status. Both physical and emotional health and well-being may be affected by the nature of the caring relationship. This may be apparent not just in terms of the tasks involved but also in relation to the lengths of time over which care giving is provided, whereby lengthy periods of providing care may exact a toll in terms of the health of the care giver as the continual and ongoing needs of the care recipient are often placed above those of the carer.

ACTIVITY 7.4

Think about the situation of a person caring for and living with an adult with a severe mental illness such as schizophrenia. Now write down specific aspects of everyday care that you think could be difficult and stressful for the care giver. Now think about this list in relation to a time-span of several decades and it is possible to see how caring might become increasingly difficult over time, especially if we consider possible deterioration in the person's condition over time as well as the development of possible health difficulties for the care giver, together with times when there could be some unpredictability in the behaviour of the care recipient.

Some of the difficulties that care givers may face are outlined in the following example.

CASE STUDY 7.2: WENDY AND TINA

Wendy was in her late thirties when her daughter Tina first became ill with mental health problems during adolescence. Tina had always been shy and somewhat withdrawn as a child, with a tendency to be rather anxious. During her teenage years, however, she became quite depressed and needed medication in order to relieve the symptoms. At this time Wendy had to provide care to ensure that Tina took her medication, that she got out of bed, ate and was generally looked after, as well as attending clinics for treatment, including

continued

psychological therapy. Following treatment, Tina's health improved and she managed to complete her schooling and went away to college. However, she found this really very stressful and was unable to continue with her course after the first term, returning home to live once again.

In the next few years, Tina had a number of part-time jobs and also further periods of depression and treatment. She also had a number of failed relationships. Another attempt to live away from home also ended in a return home, with increasing depths of depression. Wendy had to give up her work to care for and supervise Tina and found it difficult to consider that instead of growing up and leaving home to be independent it seemed that Tina was likely to live at home for an extended period as she could not cope without her mother's support and assistance. This was difficult for Wendy on an emotional level and her needs for support had to be carefully considered by the mental health team responsible for Tina's care as it was important that Wendy should be assisted to care for Tina at home.

Having looked briefly at the needs of care givers in this area, we will now move to exploring the area of abuse, adult protection and mental health.

ABUSE AND MENTAL HEALTH DIFFICULTIES

One of the problems of considering the abuse of people with mental health difficulties is that there are several definitions and, as we have seen, a number of different models concerning people with mental health problems. In addition, using the definitions of abuse, neglect and mistreatment that are available covers a very wide range of people, capacities, vulnerabilities and living situations. Moreover, there has been a lack of attention to this area within the broader consideration of adult protection, even though the *No Secrets* guidance is very clear that people with difficulties in relation to their mental health should be assisted and monitored when this proves to be necessary. It sometimes seems as if adult protection mainly refers to abuse of older people or of adults with learning disabilities but, as we shall see in this section, it also covers adults with mental health difficulties. However, although there appears to have been increasing recognition of this in recent years, the focus of consideration has been somewhat different, with much attention being paid to system-level or institutional abuse rather than situations that occur or develop in connection with people in their own homes.

This may be partly owing to the fact that, as we saw in Chapter 1, there is a long history of disquiet about institutional care and what happens to people in institutions as raised by such people as Goffman. Much of this unease has specifically related to psychiatric institutions, and indeed the anti-psychiatry movement that developed in the 1960s and 1970s was partly focused on the need for people to receive care in the community rather than in institutional (hospital) settings. Thus any discussion about abuse and adult protection in this area must take account of this backdrop, particularly since there have been a number of scandals and enquiries over the past three decades concerning abuse in mental hospitals, including Special Hospitals such as Rampton and Ashworth. In some respects, therefore, it is not surprising that some of the writing that has appeared relating to abuse and protection discusses institutional abuse (for example Copperman and McNamara, 1999; Williams and Keating, 1999). In 2001, in recognition of concerns about safety, the Department of Health produced a document entitled *Building a Safer NHS for Patients* and set up the National Patient Safety Agency (NPSA), which has responsibilities for the co-ordination of attempts to improve patient safety within the NHS in England and Wales. A central element of this role concerns the National Reporting and Learning System (NRLS), which was introduced to collate reports about incidents relating to patient safety, albeit including all areas of safety and not just those concerned with violence and abuse. However, what is perhaps a little surprising is that lessons from the results and recommendations of enquiries into care systems do not yet appear to have resulted in overall changes for individuals in hospital settings.

So for example, a report by the NPSA in the summer of 2006 that looked at safety in mental health settings considered almost 45,000 mental health incident reports up until October 2005 (NPSA, 2006). These reports were received from 77 per cent of Mental Health Trusts in England and 80 per cent of those in Wales. The majority of incidents reported, some 83 per cent, occurred in in-patient settings and 4 per cent of the reports related to accidents by patients (such as falls), aggressive or disruptive behaviour, self-harming or episodes of absconding. The NPSA estimates that, on average, an in-patient will experience 'an incident' for each sixty-five days that they spend in hospital. Whilst most of the reports indicated no or low levels of harm to individuals, 2 per cent resulted in severe harm or death. One-third of the incidents concerned mental health services for older people, including falls due to lack of supervision by staff, although the report acknowledges that older people account for less than 30 per cent of all mental health admissions. Almost a quarter of the incidents related to aggressive or disruptive behaviour (restraint techniques used, police involved, use of seclusion facilities) and just under half of the patients sampled had witnessed or experienced violence of various types on their wards. Likely reasons for this were given as illicit substance use, staff behaviours and overcrowding, with potential solutions such as environmental changes, staff training, improved patient mix and better control of substance misuse. People who use or work in mental health settings appear to be at significant risk of violence; around one in three in-patients using services has experienced threatening or violent behaviour, either from other in-patients or, perhaps rather more worryingly, from staff. The violence experienced spanned from verbal abuse and aggression to the use of weapons to threaten or attack people (although this was stated in the report to only occur 'occasionally').

The report also analysed figures of reported sexual incidents between November 2003 and September 2005 in NHS mental health settings. The report details 122 allegations relating to 'sexual safety', i.e. rape, consensual sex, exposure, sexual advances and invasive touching; perpetrators included both patients and staff members (NPSA, 2006). Significantly, none of the reported incidents was recognised as a situation of sexual or adult abuse as defined in *No Secrets* (Department of Health, 2000a). Therefore none of them was investigated under adult protection procedures. However, in addition, none of the reported incidents led to any form of criminal proceedings. Thus the report indicated that sexual safety was seen as an important issue on wards, in particular as individuals' capacity to consent can fluctuate and be variable. The use of single-sex wards and risk assessments relating specifically to sexual safety were recommended by the report in order to reduce the number of incidents that occurred.

Other central messages and recommendations from the report included the need for greater awareness of the risks of sexual vulnerability of mental health in-patients, the need for greater protection for patients, and for patients' reports of inappropriate sexual incidents to be taken seriously and appropriately investigated whenever they occur. These recommendations concerning sexual safety are similar, however, to reports from the Sainsbury Centre for Mental Health and Mental Health Act Commission National Visit Report from almost ten years earlier (Sainsbury Centre for Mental Health, 1997).

The NPSA report also acknowledged that there are areas of under-reporting from community settings and those relating to medication, clinical assessment and treatment regimes (Jackson, 2006). There is no mention in the report of the number of incidents of any type of abuse (or indeed cases) that are referred for adult protection assessment, although not all incidents would require this to take place (for example incidents relating to self-harm or abscondings). However the report does not even make mention of adult protection systems (Johnson, 2006) although some 8.6 per cent of incidents related to 'abuse by a third party' which would clearly fall within the remit of adult protection processes. Furthermore, it would appear that no further analysis was undertaken of these situations.

In many psychiatric hospitals, wards are often in need of refurbishment and the design of many in-patient wards does not appear to meet with current standards for safety. In one survey, over a third (35 per cent) of nurses in these settings stated that alarm systems were not adequate or satisfactory. The difficulties were felt in some instances to be linked to overcrowding of patients and staff shortages (Royal College of Psychiatrists, 2005). Another report considering mental health services concluded that older people could be at particular risk of violence and that many staff working with older people with mental health problems did not have satisfactory training or support in either the prevention or management of violence (Mental Health Act Commission, 2005). And as was highlighted several years earlier, the abuse of older people within mental health services was exemplified in the Rowan ward inquiry (Commission for Health Improvement, 2003; Penhale and Manthorpe, 2004).

A more recent report produced by the Commission for Healthcare Audit and Inspection (CHAI, 2006) also contained sections that considered patient safety and indicated that people with mental health problems and those with learning disabilities require more attention in terms of service provision, including in the area of patient safety. Indeed, patient safety is emphasised throughout the report, although clearly this covers all areas of safety (including, for example, infection control) and does not relate just to abuse and protection. The report stated that during 2005–6 a total of 611,000 incidents concerning patient safety, covering all NHS settings, were reported to the NRLS run by the NPSA. Although over two-thirds (69 per cent) of these incidents involved no harm to patients, a quarter (25 per cent) of incidents were said to relate to minor or minimal harm. A further 5 per cent concerned moderate harm, with no permanent effects, just under 1 per cent (0.9 per cent) involved severe and permanent harm and less than half a per cent (0.4 per cent) involved the death of a patient. Of the total number of incidents reported, however, this equates to 2,159 deaths during the year, which is a similar number to a previous National Audit Office (NAO) survey conducted in 2004–5 (before the NPSA reporting system was established), which discovered that there had been 2,181 deaths during that year and a total of some 1.3 million incidents involving the safety of patients, although 'safety' is quite widely defined, including for example healthcare-related infections (NAO, 2005). Although there is a focus in the CHAI report on the financial cost to the NHS from having to deal with patient safety incidents and their aftermath, there is also recognition of the costs to patients, which are said to include distress, injury and sometimes even death. Whilst the majority of reports made to the NPSA (71 per cent) concerned incidents that occurred in acute trusts, the second highest number (14 per cent) came from mental health trusts where, arguably, systems to record incidents are less well established than in acute trusts. However, the likelihood of under-reporting of incidents – due to the facts that the NPSA system has been in place only since the end of 2004, that there are a number of different ways in which incidents may be reported and that those incidents viewed as being 'near-misses' are generally not reported – is also accepted in the report.

The CHAI report also indicated that its investigations into allegations of 'serious failings' in the NHS (CHAI, 2006, p. 25) point to significant difficulties in such areas as mental health and learning disabilities. In these reports, 28 per cent of issues raised during investigations related to mental health settings, 10 per cent to learning disabilities and 3 per cent to combined mental health and learning disabilities settings, which in total (41 per cent) is only slightly lower than the 43 per cent of reports relating to acute settings, which are in any case much more numerous across the country. The CHAI report is clear that there is a role for that organisation in investigating local services where there are reports of serious failings in the NHS, including abuse; and, as we shall see in the next chapter, there was CHAI involvement in the recent investigation of allegations of abuse within learning disability services in Cornwall (Healthcare Commission, 2006). In this investigation significant levels of adult abuse, including emotional, physical and financial, were discovered. A further investigation of learning disability services in another NHS Trust has also been published less than six months after the Cornwall report. This report equally details situations of abuse and neglect of learning-disabled adults and unsafe practices (Healthcare Commission, 2007).

There is acknowledgement within the report of the need to 'strengthen the processes for safeguarding and protecting adults' (CHAI, 2006, p. 33) within the NHS and that healthcare services in general are not safe enough for patients. Additionally there is recognition that there is evidence of abuse and violence within some NHS services for those with mental health problems and learning disabilities and that more needs to be done in order to protect those people or patients who are most in need of support. Obviously it is hoped that appropriate and relevant links will be made in future between such bodies as NPSA, CHAI, the Healthcare Commission and adult protection systems to ensure improved levels of support and protection for those who are vulnerable, whatever this might be due to.

Abuse of adults with mental health difficulties can take many forms, as it does with other adults in other settings. It may be psychological and emotional in nature, it may be physical, sexual or due to financial and material exploitation. Mistreatment may occur as a result of neglect, inappropriate medication, restraint or other treatment. As suggested earlier, the number of adult protection reports about abuse of individuals with mental health difficulties and in mental health settings is much lower than the number of reports made about other client groups (Cambridge et al., 2006; Johnson, 2006). This may be because recognition of abuse in mental health settings has been slower in terms of publicity and identification. The impact of adult protection procedures in this area has therefore also been lower as a result (Williams and Keating, 2000; Stanley and Flynn, 2005). However, it is becoming increasingly apparent that adults with mental health problems have been exposed to both abuse and neglect whilst in supposedly 'protective' settings – i.e. hospitals – and that some abuse is perpetrated by those who are charged with providing care to vulnerable adults.

Together with increased awareness about adult abuse and protection there has also been some acknowledgement that adults with limited mental capacity are some of the most vulnerable individuals, but perhaps also some of those who are least able to attain protection via the law (Williams, 2002). Issues of mental capacity and the ability of an individual to consent to acts that may be considered abusive (by professionals if not by the individuals themselves) can be vital in determining whether abuse has occurred and establishing what action will be taken. Still, decision-making by professionals concerning mental capacity often appears to have been made on a rather ad hoc basis (Collins, 2005). However, policy guidance and legislation, such as *No Secrets* (Department of Health, 2000a), the Mental Capacity Act, 2005 (Department of Health, 2005b), and the accompanying Code of Practice, provide a framework, which is meant to both clarify and improve decision-making around capacity, particularly in relation to adult protection.

In relation to mental health, we may also find the existence of abuse by the wider community and society in terms of the inability to provide for the needs of people with mental health difficulties. As we saw earlier in the chapter, the stigma and social exclusion that adults with mental health difficulties often experience can also be viewed as abuse. This was clearly apparent in a focus group with adults with mental health problems that took place as part of the study on adult protection discussed in the last chapter (Penhale et al., 2007), in which abuse was identified as occurring as a result of the failure to allow people full participation within communities and access to services within them. Although it is relatively recently that the negative impact of society on people with mental health difficulties has been recognised, attempts to reduce the adverse impact and to promote positive outcomes need to be increased in order to eliminate and prevent this form of societal abuse for people experiencing problems relating to their mental health. And although there may not be a separate category of societal abuse within *No Secrets*, it is important that we recognise and acknowledge the views of service users themselves concerning what they consider abuse to be. We may perhaps also consider this aspect of stigma, exclusion and marginalisation as a constituent of discriminatory abuse.

As in other areas in which adults may be abused or deemed vulnerable, people with mental health problems may experience abuse:

- at an individual level – whether from self-harm or neglect or from the actions or inactions of others
- at an agency or institutional level
- as a result of social and structural factors.

Many of the interventions that may be used to assist and protect individuals with mental health difficulties who experience abuse and/or neglect are similar to those used for other service users and have been discussed in other chapters, so will not be repeated here. However, some of the more specific ways in which social workers may intervene with mental health service users can be seen in Table 7.1.

In practice, a combination of these modes of intervention will be used and the emphasis will depend on the agency in which the social worker practises. However, the

Table 7.1 Intervention and mental health

	Individual	Organisational	Societal
Statutory	approved social work assessment	through inspection and regulation	highlighting discrimination within social structure and policies
Preventive/maintenance	promoting treatment; medication compliance where appropriate; programmes of empowerment and advocacy self-management	staff development and training education for social care	campaigning for a valued workforce; appropriate rewards and conditions

fact that a social worker might be concerned primarily with individual programmes does not mean they cannot or should not take a wider perspective, highlighting evidence from their own practice to managers and taking part in social-awareness-raising activities. This is particularly important when considering abuse occurring in institutional settings and the need to bring this to the attention of relevant authorities in order to deal with the situation both for individual service users and at a systemic or structural level.

SUMMARY

In this chapter we have considered specific issues of protection and abuse as they affect people with mental health problems. This includes some of the ways in which services may contribute to abuse and with a particular focus on abuse and neglect that happens within institutional settings. Some of the ways in which social workers might intervene in such situations have also been explored.

KEY READING

Department of Health (1998c) *Modernising Mental Health Services*, London: The Stationery Office.
Department of Health (1999) *Mental Health National Service Framework*, London: The Stationery Office.
Golightley, M. (2006) *Social Work and Mental Health* (2nd edition), Exeter: Learning Matters.
Pritchard, C. (2006) *Mental Health Social Work: Evidence-based Practice*, London: Routledge.
Sayce, L. (2003) *Mental Health and Citizenship*, London: Mind Books.
Stanley, N., Manthorpe, J. and Penhale, B. (eds) (1999) *Institutional Abuse: Perspectives across the Life Course*, London: Routledge (chapters on mental health).

CHAPTER 8

LEARNING DISABILITIES

OBJECTIVES

By the end of this chapter you should:

- be able to describe social policy issues in respect of people with learning disabilities and protection

- understand how abuse may be experienced by people with learning disabilities

- be able to consider the social and family perspectives in which abuse and protection are experienced

- be able to detail a number of ways of working with people with learning disabilities where abuse and protection are issues.

INTRODUCTION

Some adults have learning disabilities, which can lead to vulnerability and a need for protection. However, by no means does having a learning disability mean that a person is more likely to require adult protection services. This can present challenges to social work practitioners and policy-makers which can be highlighted further when (developing) services for people with learning disabilities are linked to concerns about risk, vulnerability and protection. Since the publication of the CSCI and Healthcare Commission report into learning disability services in Cornwall in July 2006 (CSCI and Healthcare Commission, 2006) and in Sutton and Merton in 2007 (Healthcare Commission, 2007), and the subsequent questions asked in Parliament, the abuse of people with learning disabilities has been high on the agenda of those working in health and social care. Indeed, the announced audit of all learning disability services raises the matter still higher. This chapter first explores who are people with learning disabilities, examining some of the complexities about definitions, and then considers contemporary social work services for vulnerable adults with learning disabilities, together with an examination of risk, vulnerability, protection and abuse of adults with learning disabilities and the ways in which practitioners respond to such issues. We will also look at the particular needs of informal carers (family members and friends) and, centrally, vulnerable adults themselves who experience problems in relation to learning disability and situations of abuse. Ethical issues concerning decision-making, capacity, autonomy and the right to take risks will also be explored. We start by looking at a case study.

CASE STUDY 8.1:   JAMES

James Nicholson was fifty-five years old when the learning disability hospital he had lived in since the age of twelve was closed. Along with other residents with whom he had lived, often for many years, he was moved to a supported living environment. For many, this was to be a first step towards independence. However, James was thought to be 'too old to learn to live independently' by the care staff in the hospital and by the social worker assessing individuals before recommending a move into the community.

His parents had admitted James to hospital after a fall in which he sustained a head injury. The fall had left him shocked and stunned and he had experienced a number of epileptic seizures which had convinced his parents, and indeed hospital staff at the time, that he would need support on a long-term basis within the hospital setting. James was a bright man, well liked by current staff and someone who had taken an active role within the hospital. He especially enjoyed taking responsibility for part of the hospital grounds and worked alongside paid staff to ensure that the gardens were weeded, planted and kept in good condition.

On leaving the hospital, his notes stated that he had 'a very limited learning disability, probably compounded by his long years within the institution'. However, staff were convinced that he should not be encouraged to pursue independence and that the best thing for him would be to stay in a supported care environment. Privately, staff advised that he should not be told of possibilities for greater independence because 'he would probably pursue this but would be unable to cope'. Other staff campaigned strongly that he should be encouraged to maximise his independence as soon as possible. These two opposing views were played out without including James in consultation.

This case study is not unusual as an account of someone leaving a larger institution in the past. Unfortunately, James's experience has many resonances today. As Walmsley and Rolph (2002) point out, whilst the Mental Deficiency Act, 1913 and 1927, promoted institutional care it also set up a framework of formal care provision in which people with learning disabilities worked and were looked after in the community. In the 1980s, many of the large psychiatric and learning disability (or mental handicap as they were known) hospitals began to close. This was in line with long-established policy thinking dating from the 1957 Royal Commission proposing greater care in the community, enshrined in the minister for health Enoch Powell's blueprint for the hospitals and moves towards community care (Ministry for Health, 1962) and supported by the White Papers *Better Services for the Mentally Handicapped* (DHSS, 1971) and, more generically, *Caring for People* (Department of Health, 1989). Community alternatives were sought for people who had been cared for because of their vulnerability or specific needs or who had been made vulnerable as a result of their experiences in care with a view to maximising people's potential. In the case study above both sets of professionals think they know what is in the best interests of the service user, one seeking to continue the care in the way it was offered before and the other ostensibly acting on behalf of the rights of the service user but without consulting him. Both these perspectives place the professional in a position of power over the lives of vulnerable service users and raise questions about ethical, non-abusive practice. But both perspectives are often seen in the actions of those who work with people with learning disabilities.

WHAT IS LEARNING DISABILITY?

Terminology itself can be understood as hurtful, demeaning and abusive, and we need to bear this in mind when discussing learning disability. The terms used to describe people with learning disabilities have changed considerably over the years, but this has not gone uncontested. Indeed, the term 'learning disability' is not without its critics, who include people with conditions that might be so described, carers, professionals and others. Williams (2006), recognising the potential confusion with specific learning difficulties in the field of education, promotes the alternative term 'learning difficulties' because of the expressed preference for it by many people from self-advocacy groups (see also Emerson et al., 2005).

Part of the problem of studying the abuse of people with learning disabilities is that there is no clear definition of people with learning disabilities, and using the definitions that are available covers a very wide range of people, abilities, vulnerabilities and living situations. This, in itself, may give rise to a range of abuses of power but also allows us to understand and work with people to reduce and eradicate such abuses. Learning disability has been associated with certain levels of intelligence, notably an IQ of under 70, which applies to about 1.8 million people in the UK. However, not all of these people would come to the attention of welfare services and, indeed, some people with a higher IQ could come to the attention of helping services (see Emerson et al., 2001). Epidemiological studies in England indicate that there are approximately 160,000 adults with severe and profound learning disabilities, many living at home with their families. Also, it is suggested that about 0.5 per cent of children have a moderate to severe learning disability (Department of Health, 2002a). These figures do not, however, help us to understand what learning disability is. The importance of definitions cannot be underestimated, however, as it helps in planning and targeting services and ensuring that people who need support do not 'slip through the net'. Such functional concepts, whilst limited, are fairly widely accepted as seen in the White Paper definition (Department of Health, 2001a, p. 14) which describes a learning disability as:

Significant deficit in understanding new or complex information in learning new skills (impaired intelligence), reduced ability to cope independently (social impairment), which started before adulthood and has a lasting effect on development.

The British Institute of Learning Disabilities (BILD) considers the term 'learning disabilities' to be functional but recognises also that it is a label of convenience for planning and delivering services and stresses the centrality of seeing the person first. Using the World Health Organisation's definition, BILD considers that a person with learning disabilities:

> will have difficulties understanding, learning and remembering new things, and in generating any learning to new situations. Because of these difficulties with learning the person may have difficulties with a number of social tasks, for example communication, self-care, awareness of health and safety.
>
> (BILD, 2004, p. 2)

There are, however, a range of other definitions, as summarised by Gates (2003):

- legal concepts
- medical models
- cultural concepts
- social models.

For social workers it is the latter that are of most importance but it is crucial to be aware of other definitions, how they are used and the possible ramifications of use. This social model opines that disability derives not from any condition the individual has but from the experience of social restrictions in the environmental context in which that individual lives. As Willetts et al. (2006, p. 94) state, 'the individual's experience of being disabled is created or reinforced in each encounter with disabling barriers, and that experience is often an experience of oppression'.

ACTIVITY 8.1

Think about your own preference for terminology. Do you use 'learning disability', 'learning difficulty' or an alternative? Why do you do so, and what do you believe the possible impact of these definitions and labels might be on the people to whom they are applied?

We would agree with Williams (2006) who suggests two important factors in determining choice of terminology; first, the preference of those to whom the description would apply and, second, the social model of disability which argues for an understanding based on the disabling features of the society and environment rather than resulting from any condition in and of itself. However, we have opted for the term 'learning disability' because it acknowledges the disabling features of our current environment and society and marks a distinction with other conditions, thus preventing misunderstandings.

VALUING PEOPLE

The 1971 White Paper *Better Services for the Mentally Handicapped* (DHSS, 1971a) laid the foundations for greater in-community provision and for the closure of the large, austere hospitals that had contained so many people. The White Paper *Valuing People: A New Strategy for Learning Disability for the 21st Century* (Department of Health, 2001a) represents an attempt to continue to modernise services for people with learning disabilities. It is, in fact, the first White Paper concerning learning disability since *Better Services*. This very fact demonstrates some of the structural discriminatory abuse experienced by people with learning disabilities. The White Paper recognises that social exclusion, inconsistencies and variations in services and the organisation and operation of services may compound some of the difficulties faced by people with learning disabilities within society. It seeks, therefore, to reduce potential abuse resulting from services at both management and operational levels. It is also important for practitioners in social and health care settings to be aware of these issues.

ACTIVITY 8.2

Why do you think that thirty years passed between White Papers concerning learning disability? Are there issues for the protection of people raised by this state of affairs and what role would you have as a practitioner in addressing them?

The White Paper (Department of Health, 2001a) is based on four related principles that concur with the value base for social care workers. These are:

• civil rights
• independence
• choice
• inclusion.

The main proposals for change to achieve these principles concern the creation of integrated services by health, education and social care, and the development of advocacy services by creating partnerships with the voluntary sector. Housing and employment will be targeted. More choice and flexibility are planned. An emphasis is placed on individualised care planning and person-centred approaches to care. This will be important for individual social care practitioners who will need to negotiate change and to preserve the value base of social care. However, they also need to respond creatively and flexibly to other professions and disciplines and to the needs of people with learning disabilities. This should help to prevent the system from further abusing people with learning disabilities.

There is potential in the White Paper to protect vulnerable adults with learning disabilities by ensuring that their voices are heard and responded to and by creating single assessment and planning processes to minimise duplication and unnecessary involvement of service providers (Department of Health, 2001a). Learning Disability Partnership Boards should bring together all involved people in a locality to ensure representation. At a national level, monies will be set aside for implementation and research and a Learning Disability Task Force will advise on implementation.

CASE STUDY 8.2: LOCAL PARTNERSHIP BOARD

A local partnership board was responding to a wide and complex agenda aimed at stream-lining services, ensuring that agencies could share funding and develop multi-agency approaches to care. The inclusion of representatives with learning disabilities was welcomed by all, including the representatives themselves. However, it demanded a radical rethink of how to structure and conduct meetings and to set limited agendas that could be fully discussed, explained and understood. This led to more inclusive debate and to a greater understanding of the potential for exclusion in the development of services using complex language and closed debate.

The thrust of the White Paper concerns the protection of vulnerable people. Indeed, the executive summary of the White Paper states:

> People with learning disabilities are amongst the most vulnerable and socially excluded in our society. Very few have jobs, live in their own homes or have a choice over who cares for them. This needs to change: people with learning disabilities must no longer be marginalised or excluded.
>
> (Department of Health, 2001a, p. 2)

For the principles of the White Paper to have a positive effect in working to prevent the abuse of people with learning disabilities, there will need to be a co-ordinated response from managers, practitioners and people with learning disabilities themselves. A framework is provided but the steps towards achieving protection are not clearly articulated. And in the Cornwall report, although the White Paper is referred to throughout, there is very little mention of safety or protection in relation to the White Paper itself (Flynn, 2006).

ABUSE AND LEARNING DISABILITY

The abuse of people with learning disabilities in care settings is not a recent phenom-enon, but the definition of abuse in relation to learning disability is wide-ranging, including abuse that takes place at home and in the community at large (Brown, 1999). The term 'abuse' has been criticised as applied to people with learning disabilities, however, as either minimising the impact of serious criminal offences or sensationalising relatively minor issues. This is a point raised earlier when discussing legislation (see Chapter 3). Brown makes the important point that, however abuse may be understood, the key point is that increased awareness must lead to useful interventions in welfare services and the cultures underlying them, and to increased protection for adults with disabilities where necessary.

There have been a number of studies into the abuse of people with learning disabilities. Abuse takes place in various settings including the home, the wider community and formal institutional and care settings. The latter was brought to the fore in a number of inquiries into care and poor treatment in long-stay hospitals (DHSS, 1969; 1971b; 1972) and clearly seen again in the 1990s when the long-term abuse of residents in the Longcare homes in Buckingham came to light. This high-profile case, resulting in convictions and the suicide of the owner, Gordon Rowe, highlighted the importance of protection of people with learning disabilities. Unfortunately, the recent findings published by the Commission for Social Care Inspection and the Healthcare Commission (2006) into abuse into a hospital and group homes in Cornwall, and the subsequent call for an audit of practice in all care homes for people with learning disabilities, emphasise that much is still to be done.

Abuse takes many forms, as it does with other people in other settings. It may be physical, sexual, financial and material, it may occur as a result of neglect, inappropriate medication, restraint or other treatment and perhaps abuse by the wider community and society at large by our failures to address the needs of people with learning disabilities and in not having removed the barriers that prevent people with learning disabilities having full access to community services. The impact of society on people with learning disabilities has been recognised and attempts to address it seen in the promotion of normalisation and social role valorisation and more recently in person-centred planning.

Brown (1999) points out that, although original reports about abuse of adults with learning disabilities tended to focus on sexual abuse, it is physical abuse that actually predominates in reports where people with learning disabilities are concerned. She also emphasises that physical abuse is frequently part of other forms of abuse, whether sexual, financial, emotional or neglect. Brown and Stein (1998) studied reports of abuse under the Kent and East Sussex Adult Protection procedure in a twelve-month period. They found that 135 people with leaning disabilities were referred using the procedures, with 70 involving physical abuse and 21 compounded by other forms of abuse. Both genders were at risk but there was a peak age for people between eighteen and twenty-nine years for abuse.

In earlier research it was found that sexual abuse was generally perpetrated by men, with physical assaults being committed by a range of others such as other service users, care staff and relatives (Brown et al., 1995). In this study it was interesting and important to note that cases of domestic violence were also reported. This indicates that the range of existing ways of working with abuse in other areas may well be appropriate for people with learning disabilities and that we should keep this in mind and not create a difference, which in itself may be potentially abusive, when working with people with learning disabilities. The core difference may well be in working with care staff to ensure that they have the correct training and support to carry out their jobs, to deal with the complexities of care and to recognise and deal with situations of abuse.

In 1993, Turk and Brown published results of their incidence study of the sexual abuse of adults with learning disabilities, indicating that 1.67 persons in 100,000 may experience sexual abuse. The range of abuses included unwanted touching, verbal harassment and masturbation through to penetration, and resulted in a range of emotional and behavioural distress. Most of the perpetrators were male and known to the victims, most of whom were female. The Mental Health Foundation commissioned a project to explore the needs of men with leaning disabilities who were either sexually abusive or displayed unwanted or unacceptable sexual behaviours. The research found that, in general, 'normal' care practice let these men down. There were no key workers, written care plans or agreed channels for referral, decision-making and interventions relating to unacceptable behaviours (Brown and Thompson, 1997). It is to be hoped that under the *No Secrets* guidance these gaps will have been filled.

Concern about sexual abuse has grown as more research is completed. It is recognised that it is often more than a one-off occurrence and may involve intricate planning and preparation and even 'grooming' on the part of perpetrators. In working with people with learning disabilities the 'waters are muddied' somewhat by the intimate care tasks and responsibilities that sometimes need to be undertaken. These require careful monitoring and support. A central issue in determining abuse is whether or not the person is able to give meaningful and informed consent. Whilst, as we have seen in Chapter 3, legislation may help here, it is often more complex. Murphy and Clare (1995) suggest that there are three issues in determining consent:

- Was it enforced consent in that if it had not been given the abuse would have happened in any case?
- If consent was legal, did the person have enough understanding about sexual behaviour and the actions that were occurring?
- Was there pressure or coercion?

Of course, a further complicating factor in determining and/or working with sexual abuse and people with learning disabilities is the low expectations that wider society has concerning people's capacities, and the lack of attention to sex education and support, as noted by Brown (1999, p. 95):

> Sexual abuse of people with learning disabilities takes place against a background of negative expectations about sex. People may have little in the way of credible or reliable sex education, have few opportunities to make friends or find privacy, and are always swimming against the tide of the wish to establish an independent sexual life. . . . Unfortunately, this kind of protective veneer does not keep people safe, merely ignorant.

Financial and material abuses are also important considerations that may not be reported (Bradley and Manthorpe, 1997). The issue is complex and often concerns consent and private agreements. Consider the following case study.

CASE STUDY 8.3:   JUNE

June was forty-one years old, was unmarried, lived with her parents and worked in a local burger bar clearing tables. Her parents, both retired, looked after June's wages for her, believing it safer to do so. From her wages they took some payment for her board, bought her clothes and toiletries and gave her a small amount for bus fares and pocket money.

This arrangement could be construed in many different ways. It could be consensual and protective of June; it could be something that was imposed and abusive. It is clear that June would benefit from being involved in discussions and agreement about her wages and being helped in managing them, but the situation described is not necessarily abusive. It should warrant further discussion and investigation, however.

Whilst there is, as we have seen, a burgeoning literature concerning the abuse of people with learning disabilities, there is a paucity of corresponding research considering the effects that experiencing abuse may have on victims and their families. It may be that assumptions are made that people with learning disabilities experience abuse in similar ways to any other person. There is some merit in this argument, as to suggest otherwise may promote the view that people with learning disabilities are different and contribute to a process of 'othering' that prevents integration and erects barriers to receiving 'everyday' services. However, it is also important to consider how the experiences were perceived – similarly or differently – because of the particular experiences that people with learning disabilities have had in respect of care, in families and in the care system, and in relation to society as a whole. In this sense, the differences or otherness results from society's treatment of people with learning disabilities and not as a result of some innate difference.

O'Callaghan et al. (2003) interviewed the parents of eighteen people with severe learning disabilities who had experienced abuse to seek to understand the effects of abuse. The criteria for post-traumatic stress disorder (PTSD), changes in skills and expressions of challenging behaviour were used to organise the information. Their findings indicated that the effects were long-lasting and profound and also affected other members of the families in significant ways. This has implications for intervention and, as the authors argued, for the assessment of people when they have experienced abuse.

Hubert and Hollins (2006) undertook an ethnographic study of men living in a locked ward, finding that segregation from society leads to a loss of individual and social identity, does not recognise physical and mental health care needs and deprives individuals socially, physically and emotionally. These findings lead us to question whether some of the services provided for people with learning disabilities are not abusive in themselves. It is important also to explore emotional and behavioural issues fully for people in care or service settings. At times these may be consequential to an abusive experience and not to deal with them but to deal with the symptoms may fail the person or, sometimes, subject them to further abuse.

CASE STUDY 8.4: JIM

When Jim screamed and screamed at the lunch table, becoming aggressive if approached, some staff at his community centre wanted him to eat apart from the others or for him to be barred from the centre. Other staff looked at the lunchtime routine and recognised that this was the only time that he was separated from Rose, a friend he attended the centre with. Adjusting the seating solved the problem. If this had not been dealt with in that way but punitively towards Jim, it could have been abusive in itself.

INTERVENTION

Intervention, as we have seen in other chapters, is dependent on the ways in which welfare professionals, society as a whole and people with experiences conceptualise 'abuse'. If an act is considered to constitute a criminal act it may be that legal redress is sought or appears necessary. In the case of a welfare setting this may also result in service change and individual assistance to the person experiencing the 'abuse', whereas if the experience is considered purely in welfare terms a more therapeutic approach may be taken. O'Callaghan et al. (2003) point out that very few cases of alleged abuse against people who have learning disabilities come to court, in part reflecting the limitations of the criminal justice systems but also perhaps reflecting the way society values people with learning disabilities. Brown (1999) complains that adult protection work with people with learning disabilities is undertheorised and there is a need to build knowledge around the processes of investigation and support rather than relying on the procedural systems. When considering intervention we need to look at the process – assessment, investigation, planning and intervening – and the level of intervention – prevention, protective, responsive or ameliorative. We need also to set our framework for intervention in a context of partnership and exchange working with the person with learning disabilities or we run the risk of compounding abuse by suggesting that we know best, rather like the social worker in James's case study.

Assessment and investigation are bound with local area adult protection procedures following the *No Secrets* approach (Department of Health, 2000a). Therefore there are clear parameters as to what you are able to do and must do in certain circumstances. It is worth familiarising yourself with your local procedures.

ACTIVITY 8.3

Find your local adult protection procedure by visiting your local authority website or perhaps reading a hard copy in the local Social Services team office. They can be quite lengthy documents, so set aside an hour or two. When reading it, consider the policies and legislation on which it is built, its purpose and the agencies and professionals who might be involved. Imagine that you are a local authority social worker seconded into a community team for people with learning disabilities. Mrs O'Connell, the mother of a young woman, Jane O'Connell, who attends a college course for people with learning disabilities, has called the team as she is worried that her daughter is being pressured into giving money to another of the attenders. Mrs O'Connell is also concerned that Jane may be involved in unwanted sexual behaviour with the same attender. As you read through the procedures, write down what you would seek to do in this situation.

It appears that an allegation has been made in this case and the adult protection procedure will be invoked. If you consider what Jane's mother is saying and compare this with the definitions of abuse and vulnerability that your procedure is likely to include, you will be able to determine that the allegations are of possible abuse – material or financial, sexual and maybe also emotional. The procedures will detail the steps to take on receiving the allegation. You would no doubt, as a social worker in a community learning disability team, consult with your line manager, who will consult regarding an investigation. It may be that your team has involvement where service users with a learning disability experience abuse. If so, you might be appointed as the initial or lead assessment officer. You would want to investigate the concerns that had been raised from all parties. As with any assessment it is important to work together with the person in an open, reciprocal relationship, gaining their consent for the process and in determining risks, ways of minimising these and constructing a care plan. Accurate, detailed and formal records are required but you are able to use your skills of talking to people with learning disabilities, forming relationships and both hearing and understanding their stories. It is fundamental for this to be acknowledged in your work to prevent further potential abuse of the person at the centre of the assessment. This is also important if a strategy meeting is called to determine how best to protect the person, deal with the situation and formulate a protection and safety plan.

Where the allegations are potentially very serious and criminal charges may result, a joint investigation with the police may take place and, again, it is important that the subject of the investigation is appropriately supported. It is also necessary to know that if the police are to be involved then the full investigation cannot start until the police arrive so nobody should interview or try to take a statement or information from the vulnerable adult, as this may compromise the full investigation. Likewise, if evidence needs to be preserved for the purposes of the investigation, it is important that everyone, the individual and any staff involved, is aware of this so that evidence is not destroyed by mistake.

An important way of collecting information when making assessments stems from reminiscence work (Gibson, 2004; Atkinson, 1994) and oral history-taking. Manthorpe (1999, pp. 126–7) suggests that oral histories may help people to tell their stories relating to institutional life and experiences:

> Users' perspectives on residential services remain under-articulated and their increasing involvement in quality assurance mechanisms and inspection looks set to offer much in teaching non-users what is important and meaningful. Users' and carers' views may differ, of course, and this is now generally anticipated as a possibility. Much less is known though of

difference between users and how they may hold different understandings of residential life. Their views and experiences need to be brought centre-stage both to highlight abusive environments but also to challenge what constitutes abuse.

This approach may have value in assessment of alleged abuse. But for people telling their stories it may also have a cathartic or beneficial effect in itself. So the time spent developing a relationship during the assessment process is important and will help in identifying the individual's likes and dislikes in respect of any future work or intervention. A life-story approach may allow a service user to put into perspective aspects of their lives that have previously been ignored. Of course, for some people the telling of their own stories may be extremely traumatic and upsetting and practitioners will need to exercise caution and care. Some people do not want to talk and this must be respected. If the work is taken at the pace of the individual involved and does not try to explore areas avoided by that individual it can be a useful adjunct to communication. This method can be used in many creative ways and can assist in 'talking' to people whose skills in communication are limited. This has been recognised in working with older people with learning disabilities (Maes and Van Puyenbroeck, 2005). Pictures, photographs and objects can all be used to develop a story that has a narrative but also shares feelings, wants, needs and wishes. Stories can highlight some of the systemic and professional abuses of the past. Brady (2001) looks at the similarities between applications made to Australian courts in the 1990s for the sterilisation of women with learning disabilities and past eugenic approaches utilising the stories of those involved. This is a powerful method of work, demanding skills and qualities from the practitioner and one requiring further research and evaluation in order to develop best practice. It is a method, however, that allows full participation and for control to be retained by the person reminisicing.

Interventions that enable the person to take measures to protect themselves, to increase assertiveness and self-esteem, may be criticised as potentially blaming them for failing to stop the original abuse or as taking the responsibility away from those who perpetrated the abuse. However, skills training and individual interventions should be seen rather as increasing or maximising the potential of individuals to take control of their own lives. Not to undertake this work may in fact be more abusive by denying people the chance to develop and learn other social skills that may then open up wider opportunities. Colleges often run programmes on staying safe. Sometimes these include or are part of programmes that teach daily living skills, safety in the home and so on. Sometimes, however, they are also associated with ways of staying safe within the community. This may include walking in well-lit areas at night, letting people know where you are going and when you are likely to be back. They may teach communication and social skills that can be useful in preventing misunderstandings or avoiding conflict where it may lead to trouble and potential abuse.

ACTIVITY 8.4

Check the website for your local FE college. Look at courses designed for teaching daily living and self-help skills and assess how these might help in working with someone with a learning disability. Identify if there are any specific modules or programmes which could help in keeping people safe.

Bullying can be a problem in care and education settings for people with learning disabilities and should be explicitly addressed in a number of ways. First, it is important to assess the environment and service and to ensure that any bullying can be easily reported and dealt with sensitively. Developing an anti-bullying or anti-harassment policy is crucial in this regard. It is also important, however, to give people the skills to deal with bullying – helping to raise self-esteem, teaching people to walk away rather than react, giving space to talk (see Randall, 1997). Some local advocacy groups are now developing anti-bullying programmes for their vulnerable members.

Families of people with learning disabilities are, understandably, often protective and wish to ensure that people are not put at any risk of harm or danger. This can be especially apparent when a family member has experienced abuse. Work with families has a number of purposes. It can assist family carers in allowing certain risks to be taken but also to equip the person with skills, knowledge and strategies for staying safe. Family work is educative and supportive. Some interventions are wider than the individual and family and may involve work to enhance the awareness of staff and the safety of settings or even wider communities.

CASE STUDY 8.5:   SHEILA

Sheila had been removed from her day centre attendance by her parents. She had become quite distressed following an incident with another person attending who touched her inappropriately in a sexual way. Her parents felt this was the most responsible and protective response but Sheila herself wanted to return to the centre. A social care worker from the centre, Maureen, visited Sheila and her parents to talk through the incident and to reassure them about steps that had been taken to address what happened. Noticing the reluctance of the parents to allow Sheila to return, but also her keenness, Maureen suggested that they all attend a 'family night' that they held at the centre. The evenings were informal but supportive gatherings in which issues of safety were often high on the agenda. Families were encouraged to talk and share concerns, finding ways of resolving issues themselves. Seeing the centre and staff for themselves during these evenings, Sheila's parents were convinced that it would be positive for her to return and were able to make suggestions to staff and others about dealing with future incidents.

COURT WORK AS A WITNESS

The court system may seem to have failed people with learning disabilities who may have previously been considered to be unreliable as witnesses and unable to answer under or withstand cross-examination. Social care practitioners have an important role to play in supporting people with learning disabilities who have been abused to act as witnesses in court cases, to act as an appropriate adult when a person with a learning disability is being questioned about an alleged offence, or to support families, the police and the courts in reaching appropriate decisions in situations in which learning disability is an issue.

In 2001, the Home Office conducted a 'vulnerable witness survey' (Kitchen and Elliott, 2001), a vulnerable witness being someone under seventeen years of age, or with a physical disability mental illness, someone likely to experience particular distress because of the nature of the case or, importantly for the current chapter, a person with learning disabilities. The survey resulted from measures included in the Youth Justice and Criminal Evidence Act, 1999. Findings indicated that, whilst 64 per cent of respondents were at least fairly satisfied with the experience, the range of special measures available to support vulnerable witnesses were considered potentially very valuable.

In Scotland, many aspects of good practice in supporting vulnerable witnesses have been enshrined in the Vulnerable Witnesses (Scotland) Act, 2004, the purpose of which is to improve conditions for vulnerable witnesses and provide special measures to support them as witnesses. The definition of a vulnerable witness in this Act is widened to include any person whose evidence may be diminished by fear or distress. This is helpful in not applying specific labels to people and may be something the rest of the UK should consider adopting. However, adult protection policies and procedures resulting from *No Secrets* in England and *In Safe Hands* in Wales have led to concern to support vulnerable witnesses, although capacity, alongside age, remains a key element of the definition used:

That the witness –

(i) suffers from mental disorder within the meaning of Mental Health Act 1983, or
(ii) otherwise has a significant impairment of intelligence and social functioning.
(Youth Justice and Criminal Evidence Act, 1999, section 16)

Special measures to aid the presentation of evidence are restricted, currently, to the Crown Court, but are important in reducing the potential intimidation associated with the court system and legal process. These may include visiting the court before any hearing takes place, screening the witness from the defendant, presenting evidence by video-recording, video link or in private, removing wigs and gowns or examination of witnesses through intermediaries. The key element for social care practitioners is to support and prepare people by explaining the court process and the role of witnesses, familiarising them with the court and outlining expected behaviour.

ACTIVITY 8.5

Think of the role you might have in supporting someone with a learning disability who is required to be a witness in a case of alleged assault against him or her. What skills and knowledge would you need to fulfil this role?

SUMMARY

In this chapter we have considered specific issues of protection and abuse as they affect people with learning disabilities, including some of the ways in which services may contribute, inadvertently, to abuse and ways in which social care workers may respond to reduce and ameliorate abuse. Some of the ethical tensions involved in working in this area have been highlighted.

KEY READING

Brown, H. (1999) Abuse of people with learning disabilities: layers of concern and analysis. In N. Stanley, J. Manthorpe and B. Penhale (eds) *Institutional Abuse: Perspectives across the Life Course*, London: Routledge.

Department of Health (2001a) *Valuing People: A New Strategy for Learning Disability for the 21st Century*, London: Department of Health.

Healthcare Commission (2006) *Joint Investigation into the Provision of Services for People with Learning Disabilities at Cornwall Partnership NHS Trust*, London: Commission for Healthcare Audit and Inspection.

Marsland, D., Oakes, P., Tweddell, I. and White, C. (2006) *Abuse in Care? A Practical Guide to Protecting People with Learning Disabilities from Abuse in Residential Services*, Hull: Faculty of Health and Social Care, University of Hull.

Williams, P. (2006) *Social Work with People with Learning Difficulties*, Exeter: Learning Matters.

CHAPTER 9

LONG-TERM CONDITIONS

OBJECTIVES

By the end of this chapter you should:

- be able to describe issues concerning people with difficulties relating to long-term health conditions

- be able to detail how abuse may be experienced by people with long-term health conditions

- be able to consider the social and family perspectives in which abuse and protection are experienced

- be able to suggest a number of ways of working with people with long-term health conditions where there are issues relating to abuse and protection

INTRODUCTION

In the UK at any one time there will be a substantial number of adults who have long-term conditions relating to their health. These conditions can lead to vulnerability and a need for protection, especially at times when they have needs concerning their own safety (by their own actions or lack of actions). The range of needs of individuals with long-term health difficulties can be problematic for social care practitioners and policy-makers, given the need to consider each individual and also linked needs relating to different conditions, their prognoses and considerations of service provision. This chapter first examines what long-term health conditions encompass, including some of the issues relating to definitions. It then explores current services for adults with long-term health conditions, and this is followed by a consideration of risk, vulnerability, protection and abuse of adults with long-term health conditions. We also explore some of the ways in which practitioners can respond to such issues. We also look at the needs of informal carers (family members and friends) and the needs of adults who experience problems connected to long-term health conditions, especially where there are situations of abuse. As in earlier chapters, as part of this exploration, we need to look at some of the ethical issues relating to autonomy, capacity and the right to take risks. However, we start with a case study.

CASE STUDY 9.1: EMILY

Emily James lived alone in a small village in the countryside and was eighty-four years old when she was referred to Social Services. She had moved from a large city to live near her daughter but was relatively isolated, being 'new' to the community. She had diabetes, leg ulcers and arthritic problems, which limited her mobility: at times she was housebound. Her daughter, Linda, assisted with shopping, housework and laundry, so there was no external support apart from district nurse visits concerning her leg ulcers. One day Emily told the nurse that her daughter was stealing from her. She agreed to a visit by a social worker to assess the situation and discuss the matter further.

Emily told the social worker that she had accused her daughter of stealing from her and told her never to come near her again. She did not wish the police to be involved, nor for the social worker to contact the daughter, but she did need some help, as Linda was no longer doing the shopping and housework. Support from home care with shopping and laundry were initially provided, with some provision from meals on wheels when necessary. Routine visits from the social worker were also made in order to monitor and review the situation and to assist in obtaining local voluntary assistance with gardening and changing the locks to the property as Emily was concerned that Linda might still have a key to the cottage. Eventually Emily mended the rift with her daughter but assistance was still provided by statutory services. Over a period of time, Emily reported that their relationship, which had been difficult for many years, was much improved. Although her need for assistance did not diminish, Emily reported to the social worker that her experience of abuse was not repeated.

This case study is an account of an older person developing a vulnerability to abuse over a period of time. Although we have little information about her physical health conditions and do not know how long she had experienced these problems, it would seem likely that the combination of illnesses had probably led to her decision to move to live near her daughter so that she could obtain help if needed. The progressive nature of her conditions also meant that her mobility was affected and that she was unable to remain independent in daily tasks. Her vulnerability, which also developed, seems to be very much related to these conditions and her increasing reliance on her daughter for assistance and care. The situation that developed was probably exacerbated by the difficult relationship between mother and daughter, as this had been problematic for a long time. The provision of help and support from elsewhere (a combination of

Social Services and voluntary agencies in the local community) eased some of the tension between Emily and Linda and meant that their relationship was able to improve over a period of time.

WHAT ARE LONG-TERM CONDITIONS?

Before proceeding to discuss such issues as these further, we need to examine definitions briefly, in order to be clear about the area under discussion in this chapter. Our understanding of long-term conditions is that these are incurable and often progressive states of ill-health that can affect many different aspects of a person's life. Symptoms that relate to long-term health conditions may appear and disappear at different points in time; some will always be present, whilst others will occur for a period of time and then diminish or disappear. Although most of the conditions that we will be referring to do not have a cure and may be described as chronic conditions, owing to their long-term nature, there are often treatments and assistance that people can receive that will maintain or even improve their quality of life.

Many different types of long-term health conditions exist, such as asthma, diabetes, arthritis and neurological conditions such as multiple sclerosis, Parkinson's disease and epilepsy. Although some of these conditions (for example those that are neurological in origin) may have psychological and mental health components, it is important to note that in this chapter we are concentrating on difficulties relating to physical health as long-term mental health conditions are included in the earlier chapter on mental health difficulties. If you want further information concerning the social and health care standards for neurological long-term conditions you should read the National Service Framework (NSF) on neurological conditions on the Department of Health website. And although some conditions may be life-long and acquired at birth (for example cerebral palsy and a number of other physical disabilities) or in childhood (for example asthma), it seems that people are more likely to develop long-term conditions as they get older. In fact, one in three people in the UK and some two-thirds of people aged over seventy-five years report that they have at least one long-term condition (Department of Health, 2006c). What is also important to know is that many people, perhaps particularly older people, have more than one long-term condition and may thus be living with multiple health problems and associated difficulties, which arise from these. They can also face particular challenges, such as possible side-effects from taking a number of different types of medication and a need to see and deal with several different specialists in relation to their condition, treatment and care.

People who have long-term conditions usually have to see their GPs more often than average and are also much more likely to need to have stays in hospital at various points in time. When they are in hospital, people with such conditions often have to stay in for longer periods and are also more likely to have to return to hospital for further treatment and ongoing monitoring of their situation. Many people with such conditions need support and assistance from Social Services in order to help them to be as independent as possible. The sorts of help that may be necessary include such things as help with personal care, such as getting up and dressed in the morning, or help with washing or bathing. Specialist equipment (also known as aids to daily living) may also be required in the home. This can include items like stair rails or ramps, or specific mobility aids, in order to help people move around both inside and outside the home environment. In general, services should aim to intervene and assess conditions at as early a stage as possible in the development of the health problem. Furthermore, the management of long-term conditions should predominantly take place in the community, through a combination of social care and specialist services which are integrated at community level (Department of Health, 2007).

Some elements of the population appear to be more likely to develop and be affected by long-term conditions than others. For example, it is significantly more likely that people who live in poorer and more deprived areas will develop conditions such as asthma and respiratory problems such as chronic obstructive pulmonary disease (COPD) than those who live in more affluent areas (Commission for Healthcare Audit and Inspection, 2006). Additionally, other conditions such as diabetes and some forms of heart disease such as coronary heart disease appear to be more commonly found in particular ethnic groups. It is also possible that individuals who experience long-term conditions perhaps also experience higher levels of deprivation and this may be associated with potential societal or structural abuse, in which the abuse derives from the actions of society or the broader social structure. Such abuse may take a number of different forms, but can be linked with the experience of stigma and discrimination that people with long-term health conditions often report. As we will see later in the chapter, such perceptions appear related to a model of disability, which is premised on social aspects rather than a medical orientation. There are similarities here with discussions in Chapter 7 concerning mental health difficulties, although some of the emphases within the models are different for the different types of service user.

As stated earlier, the term 'long-term conditions' also covers neurological conditions, which primarily affect an individual's nervous system, and these can be very difficult for those affected and their families to deal with. Such conditions as traumatic brain injuries, perhaps due to events such as accidents, or stroke can have a sudden and major impact on people's lives and their ability to function. The course of the conditions may also be very difficult to predict. The person's symptoms may improve for a time and then suddenly become much worse; undoubtedly this unpredictability and uncertainty adds to the stress of the condition for both the person and their family. Recent estimates suggest that there are around 350,000 people in the UK who require help with activities of daily living owing to long-term conditions of a neurological nature (Department of Health, 2005c). In addition, however, individuals with a range of sensory impairments (relating to vision, hearing and speech) are also included within the scope of long-term conditions, as these are also likely to change and vary over time, and are often chronic in nature.

SERVICE PROVISION FOR LONG-TERM CONDITIONS

The introduction of National Service Frameworks by the Department of Health in recent years, covering a number of different conditions, has seen the development of guidance about how care should be organised and delivered for those conditions. As we have seen in earlier chapters (for example concerning mental health difficulties) the NSFs contain a number of standards that should be achieved by those who are involved in the care of individuals with such conditions (Department of Health, 1999a; 2005c). Generally, the aim of the NSF is to ensure that people receive the best possible care for their condition. This should happen irrespective of where people live or who is providing their care (whether this is primarily health or social services, for example).

It is generally acknowledged as important that services should be accessible, well structured and co-ordinated, particularly as services and assistance may be required from a number of different organisations. And, as we have seen in relation to other service users and the accepted principles of community care, care should be designed to meet the needs of the individuals (rather than fitting the person to the services that are available, as previously often seemed to be the case). As an example of this, organisations and service providers should arrange regular reviews and check-ups for individuals, in order to monitor and assess the progress of their condition(s), to ensure that the services that are provided still meet the needs of the person and that any treatment and medication that are given continue to be suitable. Such reviews can prove invaluable for the person to discuss their condition, treatment and needs for assistance and how these issues may have changed. Regular and thorough reviews can help to achieve this and to ensure that the individual is continuing to get the sort of care that meets their needs as these will be likely to change over time.

The range of services that may be required to support someone with a long-term condition will be variable, depending on the type of condition(s) that the individual has and also how this changes over time. Some conditions may be relatively stable for quite long periods of time whilst others will develop progressively and rapidly. Thus the range and type of professional assistance that the person requires will also vary depending on the specific needs of the individual at particular points in time. For instance, if the person has difficulties relating to mobility as a result of their condition (or perhaps even their condition in combination with the ageing process), then the assistance of physio-therapists is likely to be necessary to try and maintain as much independent mobility as possible. Likewise, occupational therapists may also be involved on a fairly regular basis in order to assist with physical functioning and activities of daily living, where various items and equipment may support the person living at home and help to maintain independence for as long as possible. Routine visits from district or even specialist nursing staff may also be necessary and social workers or care managers can both offer support and work with the individual to achieve appropriate and adequate co-ordination of care. Care management is likely to consist of assessment, the development of the care plan with the individual and then a process of monitoring and review, with possible periods of reassessment at times, in order to try and ensure that the care plan which has been drawn up continues to be appropriate and to meet the needs of the person and their condition. Day and respite care services may also be necessary in order to provide the individual with some outside activity and stimulation and also at times to give carers a break from care giving.

ACTIVITY 9.1

Take several minutes to think about a condition such as stroke or diabetes. Write down the sorts of needs that a person with such a condition may have at different points in time: at the beginning of the condition, perhaps at the point of diagnosis; after several years of living with the condition and at a later stage of deterioration in the condition.

Although some of the needs you have written down, for example for information and involvement in their own care, are likely to be similar at all points, there are other needs that may be quite specific and linked to a particular period or stage in the condition. Needs for emotional support may also be just as necessary as practical and physical assistance. The needs of carers will also be likely to vary at different stages and points in time. Many of the needs that you may have identified indicate some of the reasons why protection may be needed and they may also highlight some of the ways in which people may be made vulnerable or, indeed, may be abused

Access to specialist rehabilitation services may also be necessary for individuals, in order to help them to maintain (or at times to regain) quality of life. For example, following a stroke, ongoing rehabilitation over a period of several months may assist a person to regain mobility, skills in daily living (for example washing and dressing) and confidence that they are able to do things for themselves (depending on the severity of the stroke, of course). Similarly, for people with COPD, specialist pulmonary rehabilitation can help the person to continue exercising and maintain their general fitness and to overcome a fear of breathlessness which often accompanies the disease. Such specialist services can have a major effect on an individual's quality of life as they often help people to cope better with their conditions and also to make their symptoms more manageable.

Generally, people with long-term conditions want and need relevant and timely information about both their conditions and their care (Commission for Healthcare Audit and Inspection, 2006). People need to feel central to the process of their own care delivery, whether this is by management of symptoms or medication, or in other ways such as maintaining a lifestyle that is as healthy as possible (or even changing some potentially harmful aspects of lifestyle such as smoking behaviour). In order to effectively manage long-term conditions individuals require sufficient information and tools to help them to manage their own care. These are essential elements here, as are both the anticipation and the co-ordination of care needs for individuals who have chronic conditions.

Traditionally, it seemed that people were largely left to their own devices until some sort of emergency or crisis occurred and the person had to go either to their GP or perhaps more often to a hospital. The emphasis from the NSF on long-term conditions is on helping people to manage their own conditions by providing individualised care and advice, including nursing, where necessary and on providing sufficient services at the level of the local community that will help people to maintain their independence for as long as possible.

It is generally recognised that in order to achieve effective management of long-term conditions, assessment and intervention at as early a point as possible are necessary, together with co-ordination of care. Additionally, timely admission to hospital should occur when this is needed and individuals should also have access to early supported discharge from hospital, so that hospital stays are as short as possible. In order to achieve these elements, a partnership between the individual and different agencies involved in the person's care is needed. This is represented in Figure 9.1.

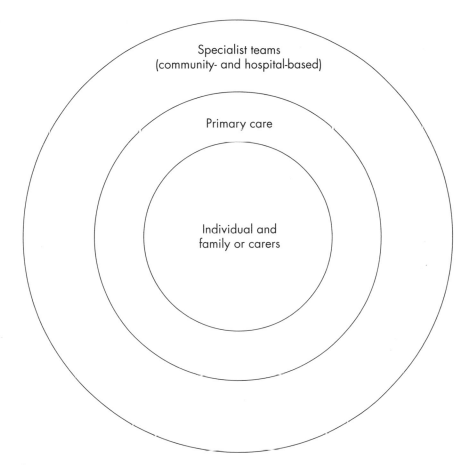

FIGURE 9.1 The levels of partnership

For the individual, the first level of support is usually their family and carers. As we saw earlier, carers themselves may have their own needs for support and assistance. In the situation of an older person with a long-term condition, it may also be the case that carers are themselves elderly and have their own health conditions. The carer will need to be supported and valued in their role within the partnership.

The second level of support comes from both primary care and local services at community level (for example, local Social Services and housing provision). This level helps to ensure that the likely problems that are linked to long-term conditions can be picked up at an early stage and dealt with at a local level through the provision of services from the locality. Further to this level is an additional, tertiary layer of support from specialist health and care services in the community. The aim here is to support the local services and to try to reduce levels of need for acute hospital care and long-term residential and nursing home services for as long as possible. However, specialist hospital services are also available at this level of support, as necessary for individuals with complex and long-term needs.

What has been presented is a somewhat idealistic model of the services that should be available and provided for those in need as they are required. However, we must also acknowledge here that services are not always available and do not always meet the needs of individuals. This has become apparent from an increasing number of service user or patient surveys about the provision of care and services. Although the NSFs provide guidance about how care should be provided and some evidence has been accruing that indicates that some improvements have been made in both the delivery and organisation of care (Commission for Healthcare Audit and Inspection, 2006), a number of patient surveys undertaken by the Commission for Healthcare Audit and Inspection as part of their review of health care indicate that the experiences of some individuals are still unsatisfactory and not positive, with people having difficulty in accessing regular reviews or specialist rehabilitation services for their conditions. For example, in recent surveys of people who have experienced strokes, many individuals did not obtain all the support that they needed, especially once they had left hospital, so whilst 87 per cent of patients rated their care from good to excellent as they left hospital, this dropped to 66 per cent a year later (Commission for Healthcare Audit and Inspection, 2006). In addition, individuals' needs were not always taken into account if they were admitted to hospital, especially if this was in relation to another or an unrelated condition. Better information about treatment and care is cited by people as a necessary component in the provision of good quality care and increased involvement of people and their carers and families is clearly also very important in relation to this.

STIGMA AND DISCRIMINATION

In the previous chapter considering mental health needs, we saw that many individuals with such difficulties consider that the discrimination, oppression and stigma caused by the attitudes of wider society are in effect abusive towards them. Views that are not dissimilar are also evident in relation to long-term conditions, particularly concerning individuals with physical disabilities. Indeed in the 1980s disability activists and academics began to discuss and develop a social model of disability, arguing that it is the ways in which society views and treats individuals with physical impairments that is disabling rather than the impairment itself (Oliver, 1983; 1990). There was a rejection of the term 'the disabled' as this implied that all people were part of the same undifferentiated group and additionally linked to views about 'normality' together with some underlying perceptions that individuals with difficulties should aim to be like the rest of 'normal' society.

Traditionally there had been a tendency to see disability as a personal tragedy for the person and their family and as an instance of individual pathology (in terms of a medical model), whereas the social model suggests strongly that it is rather this societal view that is problematic and that causes difficulties for the individual, not the condition itself (Oliver, 1990). In recent years we have seen the development of an emphasis on the need to counter discrimination, including the passing of legislation in this area (for example the Disability Discrimination Act, 1995). This does not mean, however that societal attitudes have changed totally in the time since legislation was passed, and there is arguably still a tendency for people with physical conditions and disabilities either to be marginalised and excluded from mainstream society or to be treated in a somewhat tokenistic way. It is also important to take into account the views of individuals on these issues, however, and, just as we saw in the earlier chapter concerning individuals with mental health difficulties, in the research study where focus groups were held with service users to discuss their perceptions of abuse and protection, people with disabilities raised issues concerning experiences of discrimination and social exclusion as being abusive (Penhale et al., 2007).

THE NEEDS OF CARERS OF PEOPLE WITH LONG-TERM CONDITIONS

To provide care for an individual with complex needs, in relation to individuals with long-term condition(s), can be a very demanding and exacting role. The nature of the tasks involved is such that the role may be physically very demanding, for example in the situation of a person with problems in relation to physical health or disability or of progressive neurological conditions. It may also be psychologically and emotionally demanding. The nature of care giving is such that there are likely to be both physical and mental health components to different forms of care giving and these may affect carers at particular times and for particular conditions. If a care giver has to provide full and total care in relation to an individual's physical needs and in effect to be on call twenty-four hours a day, this will be both physically tiring and emotionally wearing owing to the constant nature of the role, including periods of lack of sleep and broken nights. In addition, the unpredictable nature of many long-term conditions in terms of fluctuation, nature of symptoms and progressive but uncertain deterioration, can add to the pressures experienced by carers as well as changeability and variation in the nature of the tasks that are required in order to care for the individual appropriately.

As we saw in Chapter 7, family care givers are also likely to experience strong emotional reactions to the illness of the person they are caring for. There may be elements of loss and grief involved in relation to particular conditions, including the loss of good health and changes in the nature of the relationship as this is now based on care giving rather than intimacy. There may also be thwarted hopes and expectations, for example in the case of individuals who develop long-term conditions such as stroke or Parkinson's disease in later life, so that the period of retirement may become dominated with issues relating to health (or rather ill-health), care and treatment instead of the hoped-for development and pursuit of new activities and relationships. The fluctuation of such conditions as Parkinson's disease, in terms of the variability of symptoms and degrees to which individuals can do things for themselves, which can change quite rapidly, may also not assist a carer to cope with a situation.

Such factors as these may mean that it can be stressful for both the principal care giver and other family members to deal with. There may also be an effect on the care giver's own health. Both physical and emotional health and well-being can be affected by the nature, role and tasks associated with the caring relationship. Some carers may find care giving to be a satisfying and fulfilling role to undertake (Nolan et al., 1998). However, others may find that as the tasks involved become more complex and difficult (perhaps particularly in relation to progressive conditions) and the length of time over which care giving is provided extends, care giving is likely to become more problematic and to exact a toll in terms of the health of the care giver.

ACTIVITY 9.2

Consider the situation of a person caring for and living with an adult with a long-term condition such as stroke. Now write down specific aspects of everyday care that you think could be difficult and stressful for the care giver. Think about this list in relation to a time-span of several years, perhaps even a decade or so and it is possible to see how caring might become increasingly difficult. This may be especially apparent if we consider a likely deterioration in the person's condition over time as well as the development of possible health difficulties for the care-giver.

CASE STUDY 9.2: DAISY

Daisy Edwards was eighty-eight years old when referred to Social Services by an anonymous caller concerned about the possibility of abuse between Daisy and her husband, Arthur. Both were physically frail but managing at home; Daisy had severe osteoarthritis and consequential mobility problems and required more assistance than Arthur did; indeed Arthur had assumed a caring role for his wife and undertook some of the household tasks. Initial enquiries via the family doctor did not result in a visit by the social worker as the doctor was due to visit anyway and suggested that he should assess the situation in the first instance. Assistance from Social Services was offered to the couple by the doctor but declined at that point. Within several weeks, however a referral for support and assistance was received from the district nurse involved in the situation, with the couple's agreement.

The couple were visited by the social worker, who assessed their needs for assistance. Support for the couple was provided by regular visits from the social worker; home care assistants provided some help for Daisy, particularly with personal care. There were regular visits by the district nurse and family doctor. The local voluntary group, Crossroads, provided a sitting service to enable Arthur to go out and play bowls on a regular basis. Day care and respite care for Daisy in a local residential home were offered and refused at that point. The relationship between the couple was described as 'strained and stormy'. Arthur was very dominant and at times would not allow Daisy to answer questions; at others he could be very verbally aggressive towards her. Daisy was submissive and when interviewed separately described the marriage as difficult. She did not wish to leave the situation, however, and saw marriage as 'for ever'. Over time, as Daisy's health deteriorated, Arthur found it more difficult to cope and to provide the levels of care that were needed for Daisy. Eventually the couple agreed that regular day care and respite care should be arranged for Daisy at a local residential home. Arthur in particular was initially somewhat suspicious and very reticent, but over time was also accepting of his need for a break.

Then, suddenly, Arthur was taken ill with heart-related problems and admitted to hospital. Daisy asked for and was admitted to the residential home she was familiar with. Arthur recovered but himself needed care. He was therefore admitted to the same home as Daisy. The couple were offered shared accommodation in the home, which Daisy refused. Arthur died of a major heart attack after a period of several months in the home; Daisy continued to live there for several years and to receive the care she needed before she died.

Some of the difficulties that care givers may face are outlined in the case study above. Having looked briefly at the needs of care givers, we now explore the area of abuse, adult protection and long-term health conditions.

ABUSE AND LONG-TERM CONDITIONS

One of the problems when considering the abuse of people with long-term conditions is that, as was apparent earlier, there are several definitions of abuse and a number of different long-term conditions, so that it is not really possible or desirable to consider one single group of adults with long-term conditions. And as we have seen from the variety of definitions of abuse, neglect and mistreatment, a very wide range of people, capacities, vulnerabilities and living situations are covered. Furthermore, there has been a relative lack of attention to this area in consideration of adult protection, even although the *No Secrets* guidance is very clear that people with difficulties in relation to their physical health are included within the remit of adult protection and therefore should be assisted, monitored and their needs reviewed when this proves to be necessary (Department of Health, 2000c).

As was apparent in relation to mental health difficulties, although it appears that adult protection mainly refers to abuse of older people or of adults with learning disabilities, the term also clearly covers adults with physical health problems (Cambridge, 2006). However, although there appears to have been increasing recognition of this in recent years, the focus of consideration seems to have been somewhat different, with much attention being paid to system-level or societal abuse rather than situations that occur or develop in connection with people in their own homes. Arguably, situations of abuse that occur between individuals in the domestic setting should be considered within the purview of domestic violence. However, it would seem that domestic violence services are not necessarily able to accommodate the needs of women with disabling and/or long-term conditions and therefore needs in relation to abuse and mistreatment may not be dealt with at an appropriate level when they occur. This is where an effective and 'joined-up' multi-agency approach, with appropriate (and mutual) linkage between adult protection and domestic violence systems and services, would undoubtedly prove extremely beneficial.

Abuse of adults with long-term conditions and physical health difficulties can take many forms, as it does with other adults in other settings. It may be psychological and emotional in nature, it may be physical, sexual or owing to financial and material exploitation. It may also consist of a combination of several different types of abuse (for example, physical and psychological, financial and physical) and it is arguable that psychological abuse is always an element within abusive situations. The abuse may also occur as a result of neglect, inappropriate medication, restraint or other mistreatment, perhaps especially in institutional settings. The number of adult protection reports about abuse of individuals with physical health difficulties is lower than the number about other client groups, except that it is generally slightly higher than for individuals with mental health difficulties (Action on Elder Abuse, 2006). The following case studies may assist in indicating the range of different situations and circumstances that may arise within a consideration of long-term conditions.

CASE STUDY 9.3: DIANA

Diana Brown was seventy-six when she was admitted to hospital. She had severely ulcerated legs, was confused and dehydrated on admission, with some signs of malnutrition. She recovered slowly, and was visited irregularly by her son, with whom she lived. Diana's husband had died about ten years previously, of a heart attack, just after he retired. Her son was forty-seven years old and had always lived at home as he had never married. He had two jobs and seemed to be rarely at home for any length of time.

A home visit with Diana, prior to discharge from hospital, revealed that the house was old and in poor condition, with very little furniture and only one small electric heater to provide warmth. Diana slept on the settee in the living room where the heater was; in fact she was confined to the ground floor of the house as she could no longer get upstairs. There was very little food in the house, as her son seemed to bring in food on a meal-by-meal basis. He controlled the finances for the home and had done so for some years.

Diana said that she did not really want to return home and wished she could be somewhere where she could be looked after. From the hospital she went to a small residential home, close to where she had lived, for a period of short-term care. Whilst there she decided that she would like to stay in the home. Fortunately, a vacancy arose in the home towards the end of her period of respite, and her son was also agreeable that she should stay there. Diana settled into the home very well and lived there until her death several years later.

This situation appears to have arisen as a result of Diana's declining physical health and the generally poor conditions in which she lived. These seem to have been exacerbated by her son's behaviour and his apparent failure to provide adequate nutrition and other care for his mother. The following case study concerns a different type of situation, but also involving a mother and son.

CASE STUDY 9.4:   JOAN

Joan Wentworth was in her mid-eighties when referred to Social Services for assistance by the family doctor. She lived with her husband and unmarried son and had severe physical health problems including visual problems (blindness) and mobility problems due to arthritis and osteoporosis. She was dependent on her husband, Alfred, for assistance with most tasks. Alfred had been taken seriously ill and admitted to hospital as an emergency. Joan was in need of urgent assistance as her son was away from home at work from 6.30am to 7.30pm during the week.

Joan was provided with day care at a local residential care home during the week and home care assistance in the mornings to make sure she was up and could go to day care and in the evenings on her return from day care but before her son arrived home from work. Unfortunately, Alfred died in hospital so the temporary care arrangements became more permanent. Joan was provided with respite care at the home on a regular basis in part to provide relief for her son from caring for his mother in the evenings and at weekends.

After several months, during a review of the situation with the social worker, the son indicated that he was finding the care of his mother increasingly difficult to cope with. He talked of a number of occasions when he had locked his mother in her bedroom and in the house at weekends whilst he went shopping. The son also said that he had begun to neglect her for periods of time if he was busy with some other task. He was concerned about these situations and did not want them to continue or to escalate. Discussion with Joan determined that she too was unhappy with the situation and did not wish the pressures on her son to continue.

Following the review, admission to residential care for Joan on a permanent basis was considered necessary. Joan and her son both wished this to happen; in fact it was Joan's suggestion. Joan wanted to go to the residential home she was familiar with, so there was a wait of several months for a vacancy at that particular home. Joan settled well in the home and the relationship with her son was reported as improved at a review of Joan's placement some months later. Joan remained living in the home until her death after several years.

In this situation, Joan's son was suddenly and unexpectedly thrust into the role of care giver when his father was taken ill and died. Although local services provided some care for Joan during the week to assist the family to stay together, over a period of time it became apparent that it was not possible to maintain this in the longer term. Fortunately both Joan and her son recognised that this was the case before circumstances developed into a severely abusive situation and it was possible to avoid this through timely intervention that was acceptable to both mother and son. Although it appeared within this situation that a great deal of support was provided and that objectively this was therefore not very stressful for the son to deal with, his subjective perception was that this was very difficult for him and that he could not continue to provide care on a long-term basis. Steinmetz (1990) suggests that it is this subjective perception which is very important to attend to, for if an individual perceives a situation to be very difficult and stressful and sufficient assistance is not available to address this issue with the person then the situation could deteriorate and an abusive or neglectful situation could then develop. Certainly in Joan's situation, the son had begun to neglect his mother; fortunately he was able to raise the issue with his mother and the social worker and appropriate steps were taken to resolve the situation without a further deterioration in the circumstances.

The final case study raises a set of different issues.

CASE STUDY 9.5:   ROBERT

Robert Jackson was in his early sixties and had multiple sclerosis. Social Services and health organisations had known him for some years because of the progressive nature of his condition. He lived with his wife; this was the second marriage for both of them. No other family members lived close by as the couple had moved to the area on retirement. Robert's wife had a history of mental health problems, including several admissions to hospital when she was younger. She had a volatile temper and a rather difficult personality. She was very critical of the care and services received from health and Social Services and went through periods of 'sacking' staff who came to the home for quite minor transgressions (for example, failing to say 'good morning' in the right way on arriving).

Robert had regular periods of respite care in a local community hospital. There was much concern over a lengthy period that his wife physically abused him and, indeed, several incidents were recorded in the medical notes. There was also concern, however, about neglect of Robert. Over a period of time, his wife increasingly failed to care for him adequately. She refused to provide personal care and basic hygiene for him, but was reluctant to allow others to do this. She left him alone, locked in their bungalow and unable to summon help (the telephone was placed where he could not reach it) whilst she went out shopping. Several times he was also left without sufficient food and drink whilst she went to visit friends for the day.

Meetings, including case conferences, were held. Discussions were held with the couple about the issues and the concern for Robert's safety, but these failed to resolve the situation satisfactorily. Robert was clear that he wished to remain living at home, with his wife. She agreed to make certain changes to her behaviour and her care of Robert, but these were never sustained for any length of time. During one of his periods of respite care, Robert stated that he did not want to return home and that he wanted to be looked after properly. A place was found for him in a local nursing home, where he lived until he died three years later.

In this situation, it was clear that Robert's wife could not care for him adequately, particularly as the progressive nature of his condition meant that he deteriorated over time, but that the rate of deterioration was unpredictable. Owing to her own difficulties, she was not emotionally, practically or physically able to provide the right care for him, although it was clear that there was still a bond of affection between the couple. However, Robert retained sufficient capacity to be able to decide what he wanted and what should happen in the situation. And although it was difficult for the health and Social Services staff who were working with Robert and his wife to see the situation deteriorate and abuse and neglect occur, the approach taken, to allow Robert to remain in control of the decisions about his life and the situation, was appropriate. Indeed, much of the work in this situation revolved around offering support and supervision to the health and Social Services staff involved to enable them to deal with the stress of the situation and accept the fact that they could not easily 'fix' the problem and that Robert had the right to his autonomy.

ACTIVITY 9.3

Having read the three case studies, draw two columns on a piece of paper and list in the first column as many aspects of each case as you can that suggest possible abuse, and add a sentence stating why you think that. In the second column, identify, where you can, alternative explanations. This will help you in making assessments that take into account all the available evidence. Of course, in actual practice you would be working together with people using services and their carers, but this activity will help in thinking about assessments concerning abuse and protection.

In considering long-term conditions and abuse, we may also find the existence of abuse by the wider community and society. This is particularly evident in terms of the inability of society to provide adequately for the needs of people with physical health difficulties. As we saw earlier in the chapter, the discrimination and social exclusion that adults with long-term conditions often experience can also be perceived as abuse. And therefore the societal and systemic levels at which abuse and neglect occur are clearly very important, in particular at the level of individual experience and the impact of such situations on individuals. This may mean that there is a need to re-evaluate some of the definitions that are in use in order to allow for the inclusion of such viewpoints. As we have seen, the general definition in use in *No Secrets* is very broad:

> Abuse is the violation of an individual's human and civil rights by any other person or persons.
>
> (Department of Health, 2000c, para. 2.3)

However, the associated typology that appears in the guidance does not really allow for an adequate consideration of societal abuse, although this category is recognised in definitions that are used elsewhere, for example in France. As suggested in Chapter 7, this would appear to be necessary in the future, at least within the deconstruction and development of the category of discriminatory abuse. This lack of deliberation concerning societal abuse and adults with long-term conditions is similar to the situation relating to individuals with mental health difficulties, and this suggests that the situation should be addressed in future, perhaps initially through further research to ascertain the views of service users about such issues.

INTERNATIONAL INTERVENTIONS RELATING TO ABUSE, DISABILITY AND LONG-TERM CONDITIONS

A number of interventions have been developing throughout the world for adults, including those with long-term health conditions, who have been exposed to abuse and who require support and protection. This section summarises some of the approaches that have been taken in different international contexts. Although legislation may be considered as a form of intervention, this section will not directly consider the situation regarding specific legislation in relation to the protection of adults in other countries. In Quebec, Canada, there has been a pilot study concerning interventions, including ethical dimensions, in the area of elder abuse (Beaulieu and Leclerc, 2006) and ongoing work in the form of a large-scale study is under way. Hightower et al.'s work concerning older abused women (Hightower et al., 1999; 2002; 2006) is useful as it considers the specific needs of frail older women who have been abused. The studies have established that older women indicate that they need a safe environment, advocacy, information, emotional and peer support, which is similar to the stated needs of younger women who experience domestic violence. These findings have also been established in Australia in several projects concerning older women and abuse (Mears and Sargent, 2002; Sargent and Mears, 2002; Schaffer, 1999).

In the US, Roberto et al. (2004) examined ninety-five substantiated abuse cases concerning older women. When considering the outcomes, they discovered that 80 per cent of the victims received Adult Protective Services. Such services consisted of counselling, case management and health- and community-based services. A further 18 per cent of abused individuals were moved, primarily to residential settings. Only four of the perpetrators were prosecuted, perhaps underlining the difficulty of pursuing a criminal justice route for abusive situations. A further study considering elder sexual abuse in one US state over a five-year period determined that the most common outcome of cases was for the individual to be moved. Interestingly, this was both for victims (16 per cent) and for perpetrators (29 per cent) (Teaster and Roberto, 2004). Only four prosecutions were mounted (from ninety-five cases), although three perpetrators were eventually convicted. In this situation, only a small number of victims received either physical or psychological treatments (11 per cent); similarly, only a small number of perpetrators received psychiatric treatment (10 per cent). Reingold (2006) has reported on a programme to develop an elder abuse shelter (refuge) in New York, which combines prevention and intervention in a long-term (residential) care setting and consists of initiatives both to make the home safe and to provide a secure and high-quality refuge for individuals.

In Norway in the late 1980s, the Ulleval project was carried out to learn more about the problem of elder abuse and the extent of practical measures to respond to abuse (Hydle and Johns, 1992). The findings indicated that, although practical measures (e.g. help in the home, residential care) were available, these were not readily accessible for frail older people, for a number of reasons. Following this, the Norwegian government funded the Mangelrud Project in one district of Oslo (a three-year study), which was developed in order to assist victims to seek help and also to co-ordinate action based on the individual's needs (Johns and Juklestad, 1995). The project was successful in reaching and assisting frail older people who were at risk of abuse and this resulted in the local authority continuing (and extending) Elder Protective Services as an integrated part of the municipal services. In 1999 the model was further extended to cover the whole of Oslo's administrative districts and subsequently it has been developed in the city of Trondheim (Juklestad, 2004). Government funding has also been made available for a Norwegian Centre on Violence and Traumatic Stress Studies (formerly the National Resource Centre for Information and Studies on Violence), which is funded by several different government ministries. This centre provides information, advice and guidance for both the public and professionals. Centre staff also undertake research in a number of areas, including violence, domestic violence and sexual abuse; elder abuse and abuse against adults with disabilities are considered as part of this area (Juklestad, personal communication).

Telephone helplines have been developed in a number of different countries and serve a number of different purposes, often providing advice and information. So for example, in the UK, Action on Elder Abuse developed a helpline in 1995 as a resource for older people, their families and individuals (such as professionals) who might want to find out more about abuse or discuss, in confidence, a situation that they are concerned about and obtain advice about what they might do about the situation (Action on Elder Abuse, 2005). A Norwegian helpline was established in 2006, along the lines of the AEA model (one centralised number for the country to provide information and assistance), and early indications are that the line is used by an increasing number of frail elders (Juklestad, personal communication). Other helpline initiatives have been developing in a number of states in Australia (Kurrle, personal communication) and Japan (Tatara, personal communication) in recent years.

In France a different model of helpline is available under the auspices of the NGO ALMA ('Allo Maltraitance des Personnes Agées) (ALMA, 2004). Instead of having one central number, this service operates on the basis of separate branches in most of the different French departments (administrative districts). As is found in the model developed by Action on Elder Abuse, volunteers staff the helpline, with volunteers all receiving specialised training. The service operates with a system of referral to local services, if needed, and will also follow up cases at local level if necessary. This approach by ALMA has been replicated in Belgium, Mexico and also Italy (Casasola, 2005; Colmo, 2006).

Helplines exist also in a number of German states although there is no national strategy concerning such initiatives (Goergen, 2006). For instance, an Emergency Care telephone system was established by one state (Schleswig-Holstein) in 1999 through co-operative sponsorship. Whilst there is one central co-ordinating organisation, forty-five different organisations are involved at local level. Local complaint centres (for deficiencies in care) can also receive abuse-related complaints, and in Bonn a specialist emergency telephone line called 'action instead of abuse' receives in excess of 1,200 calls a year, predominantly from older people themselves. In 2005 the Bonn service commenced a system of home visiting (if necessary) to follow up calls; this is stated to be increasingly used (Goergen, 2006).

In the US there are also toll-free helpline numbers in most states. These are a mixture of state-run Adult Protective Services (APS) lines that receive calls about adults who have been abused and also NGO-run helplines. One example of this is a telephone line, known as the 'Senior-Info' line, in North Dakota providing advice and information on abuse (Prairie Rose, 1995). There are also statewide Senior Legal Hotlines, which exist in around twenty states. These lines provide legal advice following an initial referral call. Services such as document review, drafting of documents or referral to other longer-term services are provided. These programmes often deal with difficulties in relation to abuse and neglect (although usually not self-neglect) of older and disabled adults as a part of their remit (Wood, 2006).

In recent years there have also been a number of international initiatives to respond to the needs of younger adults with long-term conditions and disabilities who have experienced abuse. These have included initiatives relating to sexual abuse, disability and domestic violence (for example, Civjan, 2000; Sobsey, 2000; Wisseman, 2000). In one US state, Chang and colleagues undertook research to find out whether domestic violence programmes responded to the needs of women with disabilities who experienced domestic violence. The research found that although some 95 per cent of programmes did provide services for women with disabilities, there were particular difficulties in meeting the needs of this group of women. These difficulties included a lack of funding, lack of training for staff about the needs of women with disabilities and also the limitations of refuges, particularly in terms of physical space and equipment (Chang et al., 2003). In the UK, McCarthy evaluated a refuge for women with disabilities that had been set up in London. Although the refuge was mainly for women with learning disabilities, there was some provision for women with physical health conditions. This study concluded that this was a valuable, if expensive, resource for those women who needed such assistance. It also established that long-term support was essential for survivors of sexual abuse who have disabilities (McCarthy, 2000). Other interventions of potential interest concerning the protection of individuals with long-term health conditions and/or disabilities have been developed in Australia (Frohmader, 1998; Women with Disabilities Australia, 1999), the USA (Disability Services ASAP, 2000) and within Europe at EC level (METIS project, 1998). It is hoped that some of these approaches will be tried in the UK in the coming years.

SUMMARY

This chapter has provided an overview of a number of the specific issues of protection and abuse as they affect people with long-term physical health conditions. This included a consideration of some of the ways in which services and the wider society may contribute to abuse. Some of the interventions that might be used within such situations have also been discussed and explored through the use of case studies.

KEY READING

Department of Health (2005c) *The National Service Framework for Long Term Conditions*, London: Department of Health.
Department of Health (2006c) *The Expert Patient: A New Approach to Chronic Disease Management for the 21st Century*, London: Department of Health.
Department of Health (2007) *A Recipe for Care: Not a Single Ingredient*, London: Department of Health.
Oliver, M. (1983) *Social Work with Disabled People*, Basingstoke: Macmillan.
Steinmetz, S. (1990) Elder abuse: myth and reality. In T. H. Brubaker (ed.) *Family Relationships in Later Life* (2nd edition), Newbury Park, CA: Sage.

CHAPTER 10

COMMUNITY ABUSE AND ASYLUM SEEKERS

OBJECTIVES

By the end of this chapter you should:

- be able to describe ways in which the term 'community' may be understood

- be able to consider anti-oppressive and anti-discriminatory approaches to practice at a structural level

- be able to apply your understanding to disadvantaged groups such as asylum seekers and refugees

INTRODUCTION

Awareness of issues of abuse and the wide range of possible types of abuse is increasing in social and health care settings as we have noted throughout previous chapters. Much current debate within the context of social and health care focuses on individuals either experiencing or perpetrating abuse, and perhaps it is this that immediately comes to mind when we consider the need for protection. However, there remains a need for especial consideration of community-level abuse, and ways of tackling community issues. As we have seen throughout this book, the ways in which we think about vulnerability and protection are both varied and multi-layered. Whilst we might think, initially, of the individual made vulnerable by the actions or omissions of another, it is clear that certain groups and communities construct conditions of vulnerability for other people or may themselves, as a result of specific qualities they hold, experience abuse from other cultures and communities.

This chapter examines the uses of community aspects of social work within the contemporary contexts of health and social care and the role of this in working with asylum seekers and other disadvantaged groups to prevent and challenge abuse and discrimination. As well as dealing with anti-oppressive and anti-discriminatory approaches to social care practice in an over-arching way, we consider here ways in which social care workers can work alongside asylum seekers and communities to combat community abuse.

WHAT IS COMMUNITY WORK?

Community work has long been part of the wide array of social welfare in the UK. Mayo (2002) offers an understanding that seems to accord well with contemporary governmental emphases on empowerment and under-participation in the public sector (see also the Scottish Executive-funded centre on community development at http:// www. scdc.org.uk).

> Community work has generally been associated with holistic, collective, preventative and anti-discriminatory approaches to meeting social needs, based on value commitments to participation and empowerment particularly within wider communities.
>
> (Mayo, 2002, p. 159)

However, referring to Payne (1995), Mayo points up community work's politically problematic capacity for identifying inequities, discrimination and oppression that may often bring it into conflict with mainstream political ideologies. Community work has changed, in recent years, alongside social and political shifts to the current position favouring a mixed economy of welfare provision and increasing reliance on the community sector. This has tempered some of the more challenging aspects of community work which existed previously. The radical political approaches to community action need now to be seen alongside contemporary approaches to community care (Popple, 1995), but all of these are approaches that can be used in working with people in need of protection. To survive and maintain credibility, communities need to negotiate with a range of agencies and services and to form partnerships. As Mayo (2002, p. 166) states: 'Community workers need to be effective, then, at the levels of interagency work and at the levels of local and regional planning, as well as at the levels of grass roots neighbourhood work.' The term 'community' is itself contested in certain respects. In respect of community work, Mayo identified two relevant meanings – that of a shared locality or geography and that of shared interests such as cultures, identities or needs. Recently, community initiatives have been contrasted with state provision and have come to refer more to informal and voluntary initiatives and participatory approaches. There is some merit in this rather simplistic understanding when considering protection and abuse within communities. Involvement with statutory services is associated with non-negotiable, stigmatising and controlling aspects, whilst linking community initiatives with participatory and non-stigmatising, empowerment-based approaches provides important reasons for development.

ACTIVITY 10.1

Think about the term 'community' and the ways of understanding it presented above. Write a list of the various 'communities' to which you belong and indicate why they are 'communities'. Consider also the ways in which these communities may require protection or need to develop initiatives to protect themselves and their interests or to promote safety in a broad sense.

So communities have different meanings but include elements of similarity, whether through background, heritage, place or interest. One of the most obvious definitions applied to, and by, communities, is of ethnicity. This is often, however, based on visible differences or 'race' – which is itself a contested concept (Solomos and Beck, 1996). We must not forget that some communities have been excluded from the debate about oppression and discrimination because they lack more obvious differences or because some, such as colour, are seen to be more defining. For instance, Garrett (2002) highlights how Irish people have been excluded from discussions of anti-oppressive and anti-racist practice in British social work, whilst Mac an Ghail (2000) describes the racism experienced by the Irish community in Britain. Whatever the experience of the community in question, there is increasing recognition amongst public services that protection at a macro- or structural policy level is important to the range of communities in the UK, which can then work with grassroots initiatives providing preventative measures on which to build at a local level (see Figure 10.1).

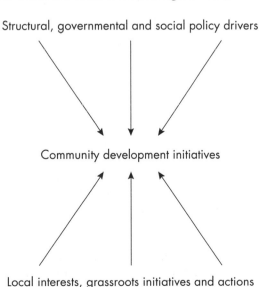

FIGURE 10.1 Local and structural drivers for community development

In Scotland, the role the police have in public protection is shown in the national 'Supporting Police, Protecting Communities' (2005) initiative which includes the necessity for all public sector and voluntary bodies to work with the police to protect individuals in their communities – in this case, where they live. After the Macpherson Report (1999) into the murder of a black teenager, Steven Lawrence, in south London, communities, as defined and organised within local authority areas, developed Community Safety Schemes or Community Safety Partnerships, with the intention of making it easier for people to report racist incidents and to deal with these across all services. These initiatives have gone further than combating racism and include dealing with abuse of many types within the community. The Bexley Community Safety Partnership, for instance, has a web page dedicated to facilitating the reporting of homophobic or transphobic abuse, to collect information and formulate an action plan to protect communities as defined by their sexualities or individuals abused in communities because of their sexuality. The website is inclusive, recognising the fear of abuse, and wanting

> to assure victims, witness [sic] or anyone reporting that they will be dealt with [sic] respect, sensitivity and in confidence. They will not make judgements about you or the crime you were a victim of, whatever your status, lesbian, gay, bisexual or transgender.
> (www.bexley.gov.uk/service/bcsp/people/homophobic/html)

This community safety scheme is focused on collecting data and facilitating the reporting of abusive incidents. This is a first step towards developing a community protection action plan. Such schemes are important for social care practitioners, as their agencies are likely to be included in the collection of data and any future development of an action plan. It is worth considering how your agency – statutory, private or voluntary – would fit into such an initiative. The fit will generally have three levels that may all be appropriate:

- strategic
- operational
- practice.

The strategic level describes the partnership in which the agency is involved, and the agreement made with the scheme concerning the agency's involvement, remit and responsibilities. It is from this strategic partnership that day-to-day matters flow. The operational aspects of the partnership concern the policies and procedures from which agency personnel work, and the practice level concerns how these translate into everyday work.

Whilst the development of Community Safety Partnerships offers a preventative approach to protection, it represents a structural level initiative, albeit implemented locally. Community responses, which can be both preventative and reactive, also represent local-level initiatives in which the community develops, determines and implements action to achieve its goals. This can also be the case when considering community protection issues. The community worker facilitates the community in responding both to its own locally set goals and to those required by social policy and governmental initiatives. This requires a range of negotiation, communication, brokerage, advocacy and challenging skills. However, the community worker is not the centre of the work but its facilitator, assisting and enabling communities to take control of actions for themselves.

CASE STUDY 10.1:   GEORGE

George was a community worker on a large postwar estate working with a group of older West Indian immigrants from the 1950s and a group of third- and fourth-generation young people. There was tension between the two groups, with the older group often feeling threatened by 'gangs of youngsters hanging around the estate' and the younger people feeling mis-understood, dejected and hopeless. Unemployment was rife amongst the younger group. George listened to both groups separately – in the community centre and on street corners – before reflecting back to them what he believed they were saying. There seemed to be a common dissatisfaction amongst the groups, a need for pride and control and a wish for identity. George then negotiated and facilitated meetings between some of the younger and older members of the community to talk and work together on ways of creating the community they wanted – creating small gardening projects, help with shopping, odd jobs and providing skills and contacts. George noted the additional benefits from sharing stories and histories of the community.

ANTI-OPPRESSIVE AND ANTI-DISCRIMINATORY PRACTICE

Anti-oppressive practice has been described as the cornerstone of ethical social work practice (Parker, 2007b). Much of the following discussion is taken from the debate concerning anti-oppressive practice and disadvantage in Parker (2007b) and applied to working in and with communities. It emphasises the relationships between individuals' interactions with the communities and agencies with which they are involved and the wider political spheres of social life. It is, however, a much maligned and misunderstood concept and an approach to social work often associated with political correctness rather than viewed as an ethical practice base. We will need to define the terms 'anti-discriminatory' and 'anti-oppressive' practice before exploring some of the implications for practice within communities.

Social care workers are often confused as to the meaning of anti-discriminatory and anti-oppressive practice. It is often asked whether the two are the same or have different and specific definitions. Thompson (2006, pp. 40–1) uses the term 'anti-discriminatory practice', describing it as follows:

An approach to social work practice which seeks to reduce, undermine or eliminate discrimination or oppression specifically in terms of challenging sexism, racism, ageism and disablism and other forms of discrimination or oppression encountered in social work. Social workers occupy positions of power and influence, and there is considerable scope for discrimination and oppression, whether this is intentional or by default. Anti-discriminatory practice is an attempt to eradicate discrimination and oppression from our own practice and challenge them in the practice of others and in the institutional structures in which we operate. In this respect it is a form of emancipatory practice.

Thompson's quotation suggests that 'anti-discriminatory' and 'anti-oppressive' practice are interchangeable terms. However, Dalrymple and Burke (1995) warn against this assumption. They state that 'anti-discriminatory practice' relates to specific challenges to certain forms of discrimination, often using legislation, such as an equal opportunities situation in which a person is disbarred from a particular occupation because of their sexuality, or using race relations legislation to ensure that minority communities' needs are taken into account in constructing community plans. 'Anti-oppressive practice', on the other hand, is taken to address wider structural issues and inequalities such as the way the organisation of society and local communities seem to favour the maintenance of the privileged roles of majority cultures and communities.

The debate is not simply a semantic one, and may be seen as having far-reaching effects on our understanding of discrimination and oppression. If you favour working solely in an anti-discriminatory way, tackling the impact of a particular form of discrimination resulting from age, gender, race and ethnicity, health status, ability or disability and so on, but ignore the impact of structural and social policy factors, you may begin to rank the different forms of discrimination in order of assumed importance or impact. A hierarchy of oppression may be created in which polarised views become entrenched and certain forms of discrimination are considered worse or more severe than others (McDonald and Coleman, 1999). This is a useful tool for those who do not wish to see change and have something to gain or protect from preserving their advantaged position. It has the potential to set one group against another without addressing core issues. Of course, this does not mean that social care practitioners should not seek to work in an anti-discriminatory way. It is important and central to ethical practice and community empowerment to challenge the focused abuse of power and exploitation of others using specific legislation, where available, and to consider the particular disadvantages resulting from a specific social division or difference. Anti-discriminatory approaches highlight disadvantage experienced by people with whom social care workers practise as the discrimination is directly related to the particular characteristics identified within the legislation. It is not peculiar to social work and social care and its operations, and applies across all sections and people within society. It is, however, an important approach to working in communities experiencing disadvantage or discrimination resulting from specific characteristics, beliefs or qualities. It is crucial for community practitioners to be well versed in social policy and social welfare legislation, empowering communities with information, advice and the means to challenge unfair discrimination and treatment.

SOME MODELS OF ANTI-OPPRESSIVE PRACTICE

An anti-oppressive approach is more encompassing. It is fundamental to set oppression and discrimination in a much wider perspective. Such an approach requires an understanding that oppression is experienced by individuals, groups and communities in diverse ways but from similar interacting elements including personal prejudices that, in turn, inform and are informed by the cultures of work and communities in which people live and forge their identities. Furthermore, these identities also interact with social factors to maintain the position of those in privileged locations in society. This is reflected in Thompson's PCS model of oppression (see Figure 10.2) in which oppression acts as the constructor of personal, cultural and societal views and is co-constructed, reinforced and revised by them as they interact and permeate the interstices of each level.

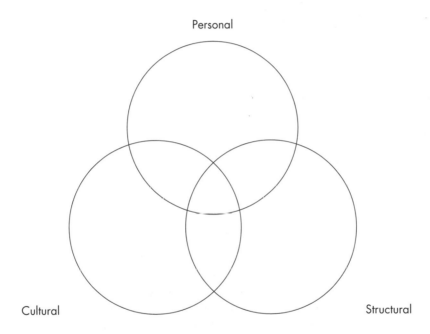

FIGURE 10.2 Thompson's PCS interactive model of oppression (see Thompson, 2006)

Thompson's model suggests that personal prejudice alone does not explain racism. It is part of it and we may all have examples of racially prejudicial comments that we have found offensive and of which we may have been guilty! However, personal prejudice feeds into and from the setting in which it develops, the living communities and neighbourhoods in which it is found, and within the schools, agencies and community groups within those locations. In turn, the way that society is organised informs how the environment operates and forms yet another influential factor in how discrimination and oppression on racial grounds develop. The personal, cultural and social aspects of life interact to create and re-create patterns of discrimination and oppression. It is important for a community or social care worker to undertake to understand this within the context of the agency in which they are working.

ACTIVITY 10.2

As a community worker you may have become aware of some of the discriminatory comments made by members of the community centre in which you work.
Since a traveller site was opened nearby, some members have been blaming the
burglaries, vandalism and perceived lack of safety within the neighbourhood
on the traveller families, having heard from others that travellers are dishonest and
having this view reinforced by the local press who provided stories and pictures
of squalor, which you later found out were library pictures of other sites. You find
that there is no evidence that the traveller families have contributed to increased
crime and, indeed, you have been working with them to negotiate environmental
and education services with the local authority. The members of the community
centre want your help in orchestrating a campaign to close the site. What do
you do in this situation and how might your knowledge of anti-discriminatory and
anti-oppressive practice help you?

This situation raises some dilemmas, as the community seems to be mobilising to take
action itself. However, this action is discriminatory against another group and is based
on prejudice, some of which is personal, some fuelled by prejudice from other agencies
and media, and, no doubt, exacerbated further by the lack of provision for and
recognition of non-static lifestyles at policy level. Understanding the ways in which
oppression and discrimination develop can help you comprehend how this situation may
have come about. You will need to use all your skills of negotiation, challenging and
presenting information to work with this situation, seeking to bring groups together to
work on common needs and goals.

Dominelli (2002) understands oppression as a continuum running from
oppression and exploitation through to empowerment and emancipation that fits well
with community development approaches. Before reaching the positive outcome of
empowerment, those who are oppressed will resist, and it is in this resistance that social
care and community workers can be effective in enabling people to challenge, campaign
and change. In order to do this, practitioners need to understand that oppression takes
place within the social arena, and is (re-)created by interactions between people in
society. Community social workers are important in working with people to reduce and
eradicate oppression because they work with people in context. However, they are also
part of society and are involved in the interactions that create, recreate or resist
oppression and, therefore, need continually to reflect on their position. As Dominelli
(2002, p. 36) states:

> Anti-oppressive practice addresses the whole person and enables a practi-
> tioner to relate to his or her client's social context in a way that takes account
> of the 'allocative and authoritative resources' that both the practitioner
> and the client bring to the relationship. Thus, anti-oppressive practice takes
> on board personal, institutional, cultural and economic issues and examines
> how these impinge on individuals' behaviour and opportunities to develop
> their full potential as persons living within collective entities.

A mystique has grown up around the terms, which has led some care workers not to question or challenge thinking and actions in a critical and reflective way for fear of appearing oppressive or discriminatory. This can lead to the very situations that anti-oppressive and anti-discriminatory practice seek to reduce or eradicate. It is important for social workers to question why things are the way they are and the impact this has on practice, on agency ethos and on the people with whom social workers practise. For instance, consider the following example.

ACTIVITY 10.3

As a practitioner working with a Guinean refugee community you are aware that female circumcision is considered by some in the community as an integral part of the culture. When you challenge this practice as abusive, a fellow worker suggests you are being oppressive as this is a cultural rite. How would you answer this criticism?

As a model, anti-oppressive practice provides a way of conceptualising and working with people in a critical and ethical manner, taking issue with popular assumptions and beliefs. It requires social workers to examine their own beliefs and assumptions and those of their agencies and wider society, and can be extended by agencies and social work supervisors to examine why these associations are made. Practising anti-oppressively is not easy, however.

Anti-oppressive practice is also associated in popular thought with popular and pejorative versions of political correctness, as noted above. This creates a conceptual, theoretical and practice base against which social workers can be judged and which may push them into socially constructed positions of disadvantage. However, anti-oppressive practice is multi-dimensional. It is practice that requires social workers to act in ways that first do not oppress and ultimately empower those individuals and communities with whom they work. It is also practice which seeks to change systems that uphold the status quo at the expense of service users, carers or people disadvantaged or marginalised because of social divisions, statuses and socially ascribed roles and attributes. A semantic issue arises with the term 'anti-oppressive practice' in respect of its negative prefix. However, whilst challenge and struggle are important aspects of acting anti-oppressively, the objective is to establish non-oppressive enabling and empowering social care work practices.

Cultural competence stems from an anti-oppressive approach to practice and concerns the competence and understanding to work with diverse groups, respecting and acknowledging difference whilst working with people to effect changes that have been agreed and negotiated together. It depends on a practice that takes its lead from the people with whom the social care practitioner is working, and a consideration of group similarities can be useful in determining the characteristics of communities that you are working with as long as you do not impose stereotypes and untested assumptions of how the group 'ought' to behave. We must, as noted by Doel and Shardlow (2005), acknowledge that notions of difference and diversity shift according to time and context and are not rigid, that stereotypes may reflect commonly observed phenomena but not what happens in every case. However, it is an important concept when working with communities and individuals in communities who are vulnerable, disadvantaged or in need of protection.

WORKING WITH ASYLUM SEEKER AND REFUGEE COMMUNITIES

Social work's concern with asylum seekers in the UK is most apparent when considering asylum-seeking children and unaccompanied minors (Kidane, 2001a; 2001b; Rutter, 2001; Torode et al., 2001; Cemlyn and Briskman, 2003). This focus is understandable given the emphasis on child welfare and protection but must not detract from the needs of adult asylum seekers and refugees, although, as we shall see later, Hayes (2005) draws our attention to this deficit in social care thinking and practice. Indeed, when establishing themselves in communities many asylum seeker families comprise adults and children. The psychological and social needs of asylum seekers and refugees are well rehearsed in the literature (Parker, 2000; Weaver and Burns, 2001), but the need for safe communities is perhaps not addressed with the same urgency. Similar trends are seen in respect of traveller families and communities, in which the place of social welfare is questioned (Cemlyn and Briskman, 2003).

Nomme Russell and White (2002) report on an educational initiative designed to include practitioners and service users of varied cultural backgrounds when exploring cultural perceptions and anti-oppressive practice. This is helpful in relation to individual understanding and practice, but there is a need to address the wider aspects of agency and community provision and community engagement as a means of facilitating learning and co-operation between interest groups or living groups within geographical communities.

Social care practice must address the wider issue of community engagement, development and work if the important, but not exclusive, intra- and interpersonal social work is not to become oppressive or abusive in itself. What does this mean? There is a danger that social care work as practised by statutory agencies may address crucial issues of individual protection and family and social regulation but, without an understanding of cultural variations and a corresponding approach to working with communities and in communities to foster wider understanding, this runs the risk of simply controlling rather than enabling and assisting people to take control of their own lives and communities. So, as in all adult protection work, there are three levels:

- a socio-political level
- a community and agency-based level
- an individual practice and practitioner level.

ACTIVITY 10.4

Think of the agencies that are engaged in community work in an area you know. List the ways in which these agencies offer culturally competent work with communities and the ways in which they offer a service that meets majority needs. How might these agencies best serve the interests of asylum seeker and refugee communities?

Highlighting social need has been a fundamental aspect of welfare since its formal beginnings in the charitable and philanthropic societies of Victorian Britain, and especially in the social surveys of Charles Booth and Seebohm Rowntree (Payne, 2005). This is no less the case today, and this is particularly important in dealing with community need. Given the changing landscape of communities responding to migration for a host of reasons, an important role for community workers is to profile the community and consider the needs of those groups comprising it.

ACTIVITY 10.5

Taking the community that you considered in the previous activity, think of ways you might undertake a profile of that community. Whom would you talk to and involve? How might you ensure that you collect appropriate information from all sources?

You would, of course, need to have a good knowledge of the resources available in the area and whom they are designed to serve, but this in itself does not provide a full profile of the area. You will need to consider demographic information to gain a perspective of the make-up of the area but also to talk with community leaders from different sections and ensure you are open to accepting minority views. This demands the use of a range of skills.

Hayes (2005) recognises the complicity of social work in dealing with asylum seekers and others subject to immigration controls according to the stereotypes and images rife in society, acknowledging that this may also lead to oppression and discrimination. She calls for the integration of asylum and immigration issues into the social work curriculum. Hayes believes that the control of welfare is important in understanding this – the idea that public resources are not 'squandered' on the 'wrong' people. This view rests on taken-for-granted ideas of who deserves welfare and a perception that incomers incur costs without recognition or acknowledgement of any potential benefits or contributions brought. Referring to social work within the contemporary social security and welfare systems, Hayes (2005, p. 189) points out:

What we now have, therefore, unashamedly, is a 'welfare' scheme, deliberately separate and inferior, making no attempt to even offer subsistence-level support and which manages and moves human beings without offering any choice or indeed any consideration of individual need. As a profession, social work is now part of that machinery administering this system. In local authority Asylum Teams which sort out accommodation, money, vouchers, GPs, schooling and so on, there is little room for more in-depth practical or emotional help for this vulnerable group. Having separated them from the normal welfare arrangements and mainstream services, social workers are operating in a system which discriminates, excludes and fuels a climate of hostility.

This reminds us that we face a conundrum as social care practitioners working within existing social policies and legislation and on behalf of those who are dispossessed, vulnerable and disenfranchised. It indicates the need for community-based and community-driven initiatives and for a robust practice based squarely on anti-oppressive values. In statutory social work teams this needs to be acknowledged, but the new culture of voluntary agency work and the funding streams that support it means that practitioners are not immune from some of the uncritical attitudes and discriminatory service provisions seen in the statutory sector.

Khan (2003) points out, by using an example from Canada, that services developed to assist people and asylum seeker and refugee communities may experience difficulties in working together to meet the needs of asylum seekers at times of immediate need. Fuelled by negative media portrayals of asylum seekers, misinformation and public fear, this difficulty can create problems for those seeking asylum. He calls for greater co-ordination between agencies and understanding of each other's particular remit, which can be achieved by joint meetings, consultation and joint training.

ACTIVITY 10.6

Consider the following example. The area you are working in has recently taken in a number of South Asian asylum seekers. This community has a range of health, social and education needs but there does not appear to be a co-ordinated approach to planning or delivering services and some of the agencies are duplicating them. A member of the community has complained to you about the difficulties of negotiating this system and has sought your help to co-ordinate ways of delivering services to this community. What would you seek to do?

BOX 10.1   A BRIEF OUTLINE OF IMMIGRATION AND ASYLUM SEEKING IN THE UK

It is worth rehearsing recent history in respect of immigration and asylum seeking. Immigration has been a fiercely debated topic in the UK since the dissolution of colonial power. The encouragement of economic immigration in the 1950s, the response to trauma and disaster in former colonies and the rising panic created by the media and some politicians have continued to fuel public debate and the development of socially constructed responses to immigration. These responses are often popularised manifestations of racism.

The increase in the number of asylum seekers and refugees has reshaped the topography of migration in Europe (Castles and Miller, 1998). In the UK this has been responded to by the passing and implementation of increasingly draconian measures to limit, control and regulate people without a corresponding concern for the welfare and protection of both individuals and groups. The increasing demand for local authority services, including Social Services and housing and other welfare agencies, to support the needs of those seeking asylum requires social workers to be educated and prepared to meet the special needs of those seeking asylum. As Hayes (2005) argues, social workers in the UK must be well versed in matters of migration, family and identity and integrate their knowledge with care management, mental health and child care or family support practice. Councils with Social Services Responsibilities (CSSRs) are often unprepared for the construction and delivery of appropriate Social Services for persons seeking asylum. There has been a range of responses to immigration into Britain, from assimilation to repatriation (Dominelli, 1997). This has come to the fore more recently in the launch of the government's Commission for Integration and Cohesion that argues again for a shift from multiculturalism to a more homogeneous society.

Immigration has characterised the entire history of the British Isles (Panayi, 1999). Mason (1995, p. 23) is clear about the historical importance of migration for the formation of the present-day British population:

> Britain's population is one forged from successful historical migrations. In this respect it is not unique, although the geographical isolation conferred by island status probably helped to make those migrations more palpable. The early phases of industrialization gave new impetus to inward migration . . . Each successive phase of industrial change and developments has been, in its turn, associated with new patterns of internal and international migration.

Early history in the UK concerns migration, invasion and settlement. From 1066 until 1915 there was continuous but small-scale immigration into Britain with much migration centred on slavery. The development of industrial capitalism during the Industrial Revolution gave rise ultimately to momentous patterns of migration, internal and external (Kumar, 1978). Migration from Ireland increased because of internal pressures in Ireland and growing labour force needs in Britain. Irish immigration has remained an important source of labour for the British economy. In between the First and Second World Wars immigration to Britain declined sharply and was largely confined to people escaping persecution, including Jewish people and continued Irish immigration.

continued

After the Second World War there was a change in economic circumstances and a shift in immigration patterns from the New Commonwealth – people from the countries of the former British Empire. This period is characterised by increasingly harsh controls on immigration in response to popular fears, hostility and racism.

The period following the end of the Second World War has also seen the development and introduction of legislation aimed at countering discrimination experienced by ethnic groups. In 1965 the first Race Relations Act was passed which outlawed discrimination in public places. In 1968 this was extended to the arenas of housing and employment. The longest-lasting piece of Race Relations legislation was passed in 1976 and revised in 2000. This Act introduced the concept of 'indirect discrimination' which applies to public services.

Consider the following case studies, thinking about what needs for protection arise for individuals and/or communities and how an anti-oppressive approach to work may assist in enabling and empowering those involved.

CASE STUDY 10.2: AHMED

Ahmed was seventeen years old, and came to the UK four years ago from Afghanistan with his father and brother, claiming asylum as they stated they were prone to persecution and threat if they remained. Ahmed has experienced substantial harassment from the white community where he lives, with taunts to return home, insults and threats to his safety. Ahmed's father was a GP in Afghanistan. He has not been able to gain a position in the UK and is working as a care worker in a local community centre for older people. Ahmed's family are living in a predominantly white British area. The families in the area do not speak to them and there have been instances of racist graffiti written on their walls and excrement posted through their letterbox.

CASE STUDY 10.3: ANTI-TERROR LEGISLATION AND COMMUNITIES

The mainly Muslim community in the area in which you work has experienced a significant rise in the number of police investigations and raids on homes under anti-terrorist legislation. No charges have come about. The community feel aggrieved and many of the younger men in the community want to take direct action against the police. A community leader has complained to a local councillor about the Social Services provided by the local Council with Social Services Responsibility, who have informed him that, because of costs, services are geared to the needs of the majority and Halal foods are not served in day centres because so many Muslims are well supported in their own community.

CASE STUDY 10.4: TRAVELLER COMMUNITY

A traveller community on a non-statutory site is campaigning for water and septic tank services. Some members of the local sedentary community are organising against the development of this site, and there has been an incident in which sewage was tipped out across the camp and chemical toilets smashed.

Points to keep in mind:

- Listen to everyone involved, collect all views
- Reflect back your understandings to ensure you have understood people from all positions
- Find out as much as you can about the area, resources and communities involved
- Ask about cultural beliefs and needs but do not assume they are shared in the same way by every member of the community; this may mean that you have to ask a range of individuals about their needs
- Challenge discrimination and unfair treatment
- Negotiate, enable people to take control of their lives and achieve their own goals.

You may wish to construct a culturagram with the people you are working with, as this can provide a powerful tool in which people can participate in providing information about themselves, their wants and their wishes (Congress, 1994; Parker and Bradley, 2003). Culturagrams are a visual representation of culturally specific information that have been used in working in adult protection to help ensure that practitioners listen to and respect individual aspects of culture and belief in planning and implementing services (Brownell, 1997). They can be used effectively in the assessment process (see Chapter 7) and in forming appropriate working relationships when working with diverse cultures and communities. An example of a culturagram is shown in Figure 10.3.

SUMMARY

In this chapter we have considered the importance of community work in protecting people and responding to abuse. Communities were understood as relating to the geographical location in which people live and as groups of interested people or those sharing particular qualities. Some of the ways in which communities are abused and in need of protection and how communities may abuse its members or those of other groups have been considered. In particular, we considered issues arising from working with asylum seeker and refugee groups.

As we noted, discrimination, stigma and disadvantage are widespread when dealing with asylum seeker, refugee and minority ethnic groups. A social care

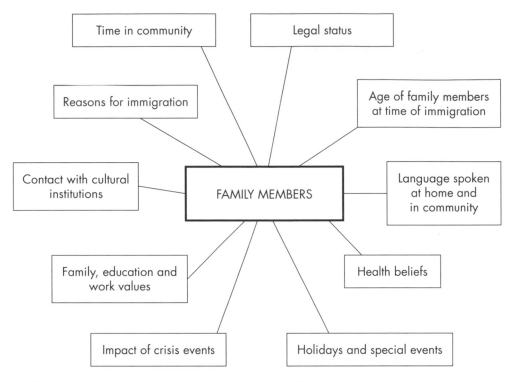

FIGURE 10.3 Culturagram (after Parker and Bradley, 2003)

practitioner working in a particularly disadvantaged area with high rates of crime, violence, family breakdown, unemployment and disease may empathise with the people with whom he or she works. Because of this, the community or social worker may assume, in the eyes of others, the mantle of disadvantage experienced by service users (Parker, 2007b). The ability to empathise is key to developing a culturally competent and anti-oppressive approach that seeks to understand the perspective of those involved whilst challenging abuses of power.

KEY READING

Cemlyn, S. and Briskman, L. (2003) Asylum, children's rights and social work, *Child and Family Social Work*, 8, 163–78.

Hayes, D. and Humphries, B. (2004) *Social Work, Immigration and Asylum*, London: Jessica Kingsley Publishers.

Popple, K. (1995) *Analysing Community Work: Its Theory and Practice*, Buckingham: Open University Press.

Tett, L. (2006) *Community Education: Lifelong Learning and Social Inclusion*, Edinburgh: Dunedin Academic Press.

Thompson, N. (2006) *Anti Discriminatory Practice* (4th edition), Basingstoke: Palgrave.

CONCLUSION

In the concluding section of the book we draw together the implications of the exploration we have undertaken in earlier chapters. We will also suggest some potential ways forward in improving the quality and effectiveness of responses to the abuse of vulnerable adults. In order to do this, we need to consider the training, supervision and support needs of staff, as well as management processes and social support. Prior to this, however, we need to briefly recap the content of earlier chapters.

UNDERSTANDING PROTECTION AND VULNERABLE ADULTS

In the first four chapters, we set the scene and context for understanding social care work with adults in need of protection. We also introduced some core knowledge and principles concerning the ways in which vulnerability, harm, abuse and protection are conceptualised and theorised. This context provides the base from which we can consider social work and social care's value base and the contribution of these to work in adult protection. We also explored issues relating to care settings of various types. However, in order to really appreciate the context and the value base, we needed to consider the legislation and policy context in which social work is practised and in particular those aspects and elements of relevance to the field of adult protection. The new alliances and organisational settings in which social work and social care are now located also warranted some examination. In respect of this we discussed the range of roles, settings and working arrangements which have arisen over recent years. Within this context, we have seen the development of an increased emphasis on improving the quality of service provision for those individuals who are in need of support and assistance from care services. This has also resulted in a range of regulation, inspection and monitoring arrangements that have been created both as a way of driving up standards and improving quality and also ensuring that sufficient attention is paid to quality issues by way of systems to monitor and review these. The development of performance management, regulatory processes and monitoring were therefore also considered in the final chapter of the first section of the book with caveats attached that acknowledged some of the potential difficulties arising from a managerialist approach to care.

WORKING IN ADULT PROTECTION

The experience of adults who have been abused or are in need of protection is of central concern to the development of social care work that is both effective and ethical. Whilst research in the UK in these areas remains limited, there is a growing body of knowledge that contributes to our understanding and to the development of ways in which we work. Chapters 5–10 were more directly concerned with practice in contemporary social work and social care and with those individuals who may require protection. Although Chapters 5–6 considered quite generic issues relating to assessment and working collaboratively in adult protection, subsequent chapters developed an exploration of protection issues for adults with mental health problems, learning disabilities, long-term conditions and the wider issue of community-level abuse. This was achieved in each chapter following a consideration of the issues involved in slightly more general terms for service users.

ETHICAL PRACTICE

When we are considering the issue of safety and protection for adult service users who may require assistance, support and protection, some common themes and issues emerge, which have appeared consistently throughout this book. One of these has been the issue of ethical practice; practice with individuals, families and even groups of individuals that is respectful, acknowledges difference, attends to cultural issues and seeks to keep the views of people who use social services central to the endeavour that is social work and social care, especially as this relates to adult protection. Together with a real desire to increase the quality of services is a steadfast ambition to really empower users of services within social care. In order to do this it is important to seek the views of the individuals involved at every point in the process and to really keep those views in focus – that is, to incorporate those views in the planning, implementation, review and monitoring of service provision. This applies within the area of adult protection as much as it does in other aspects of social care, so that the need to afford safety and protection to those individuals who may be in need of such support is also recognised as fundamental. What is also crucial here is that individuals, together with their needs, views and perceptions, are kept in a central position and not in some more peripheral position. This includes the involvement of individuals in a meaningful way in consultation and the development of processes and in the operation of Adult Protection Committees or Adult Safeguarding Boards.

DIFFERENT TYPES OF ABUSE, DIFFERING INTERVENTIONS

As we have seen, abuse, violence and neglect take a number of different forms and clearly affect different individuals in differing ways and ways that may be dynamic and change over time. This depends on a number of factors, including the type of abuse that is occurring, the length of time over which the abuse takes place (whether it is part of a pattern or not) and both the frequency and severity of the abuse. In addition, the location or setting in which the abuse occurs is of importance, as we have seen that there are differences for example between a situation that occurs in an individual's own home in an isolated setting and incidents that occur in residential or nursing homes. Further to this is the question of who is perpetrating the abuse. In earlier chapters, it became clear that there are a variety of potential perpetrators of abuse, and unfortunately this also includes paid care workers and professionals, who arguably have a duty of care to protect and safeguard an individual who is vulnerable.

The characteristics of the individuals themselves will also have a major influence in terms of the effect of the situation, as they include the person's prior experience, coping strategies and resilience, both mental and physical, to withstand, deal with and survive the situation. Intervening in situations of abuse, violence and neglect requires an exploration of these and other factors in order to try to determine the most appropriate way of responding given the individual (or individuals, in institutional settings) and in light of their particular circumstances and location at the time. Furthermore, it is not possible at present to say with certainty which interventions are most effective for which situations and types of abuse. Although some work has been undertaken in this area, and some early studies have been conducted, we are not far enough forward in terms of the overall situation to be able to sure about this. As the eminent American geriatrician and academic researcher Mark Lachs has stated (personal communication):

> Such studies as exist are for the most part observational and of variable (but increasing) quality. I am pretty skeptical that you'll find any elder abuse intervention, embedded in protective services or otherwise, that meets even modest evidence standards for effectiveness (e.g., randomization, explicit description of a reproducible intervention, discrete and sensible endpoints, dealing with attrition, etc.). The child protective people have been doing this here for nearly 50 years and we're only now starting to see quality data on some of their interventions, like family preservation.

Although Lachs was commenting on the situation concerning the USA and specifically relating to elder abuse, we have seen throughout this book that in many respects the USA has been in the forefront of developments in adult protection, with the early development of Adult Protective Services from the early 1980s and consistent research in this area since that time. If the USA is not yet in a position to determine the effectiveness of interventions and outcomes for individuals who have experienced abuse, we should not be too surprised that this does not appear to have occurred anywhere else either.

However, clearly this does not mean that we should wait for such developments before taking action about situations. Where an individual is in need of assistance, support or protection then those who are involved with the person need to work with them, taking into account the factors discussed above and the individual's circumstances and then assist in developing the most appropriate care plan which will best suit their needs. In addition, we would not in any case like to see the development of formulaic responses to individuals along the lines of 'X has happened therefore Y must follow' as this would not really be likely to take into account the individual's needs as a unique individual. There is also an apparent danger that homogeneous responses could result, in which people are treated exactly the same, irrespective of their individual needs. This is not to argue against establishing which interventions and responses are most effective, but to caution against seeing these as some sort of panacea or 'holy grail'. In our view, such information (on effectiveness) should in due course be added into the mix of information obtained from careful, sensitive and thorough assessment processes at the point of developing the care plan. It may not, however, be the predominant factor in the determination of the care and safety (or even the full protection) plan.

In addition, there is a need for more work to be done concerning the range of interventions that are available to assist individuals who experience abuse, violence and neglect. For example, if the ultimate sanction relating to institutional abuse and neglect is the closure of that establishment, which requires removal and relocation of residents, this may act as a powerful disincentive for organisations such as health and Social Services, at local level, to proceed with this action. Such a response will require much time and effort to find alternatives and to effect both the closure of the home and the relocation of residents. This may arguably not be in the best interests of some residents who may not have been directly affected by the abuse but will be obviously affected by the closure and the enforced move that they have to undertake. The use of 'trouble-shooting' managers to move into a failing home and replace a poor or ineffectual manager and avoid closure and relocation is not, however, widely used, although its use was suggested some years ago (Bennett et al., 1997). However, the amount of time and effort required should not be used as an excuse for action not being taken to close a home that is clearly failing. Closure is particularly likely to be necessary if it appears to be beyond the means of the current owners and management to rectify the situation and bring about the necessary changes within the home in order to ensure that residents are not placed at further risk of harm. As a further example, in our view, the use of family therapy for older adults and those with disabilities is worthy of further consideration and development, perhaps particularly in families where there are caring responsibilities as well as normal familial expectations. Increased systems of social support for individuals also merit further growth, particularly in relation to support groups for victims and survivors, whether these are self-help or victim support groups.

In recent years we have also seen the development of MAPPA (Multi-Agency Public Protection Arrangements) and MARAC (Multi-Agency Risk Assessment Conference) processes and specialist Domestic Abuse or Domestic Violence Projects, in which specialist multi-agency teams have been set up in local areas in response to situations of domestic violence (principally of young women). As such initiatives become more established in different areas, they are also worthy of some attention in order to consider whether such processes might be successfully adapted for work within adult protection.

EDUCATION AND TRAINING

In order to achieve necessary changes and expansion of responses to abuse, violence and neglect, however, it will be necessary to develop both the resource base and the skill base for practitioners working in this area. This will require improvements in both education and training systems, especially at the level of training for existing staff. Training in interventions should be very much part of the multi-agency training strategy which is drawn up at local level, beyond the level of those early stages of investigation and assessment, and should include such aspects as disclosure interviews, which are developing as specialised modules across the country for staff involved in investigations. That such training should be multi-agency is generally accepted, but clearly such initiatives and the development of different levels of training modules, from awareness raising through to longer-term work with individuals who have experienced abuse and neglect and intervening in abusive situations beyond the investigative stage, have resource implications at local levels.

Since training appears to be a seemingly never-ending process, with a constant need for updating and refresher training, in addition to the need to ensure that new employees who will be working in adult care receive at least some basic awareness raising training at the point of induction or as soon as possible afterwards, there are likely to be continual and continuing resource implications at local level. This is where multi-agency, jointly funded training is clearly highly beneficial, with all relevant agencies taking some responsibility and providing some financial support for training. Unfortunately, however, this is not yet found as a standard approach to the provision of adult protection across the country, so that, whilst multi-agency training exists, funding for this may not be shared. This may be for a number of reasons, including a lack of resources and infrastructure at local levels to allow for this within organisations (Perkins et al., 2007).

It also appears that education at pre- and post-qualifying levels, to prepare professionals for the world of human services, means that students have to acquire proficiency in interpersonal and communication skills and also develop skills in engaging with individuals in difficult, stressful and sensitive situations, including those which concern abuse, violence and neglect. This will additionally require the development of knowledge and understanding of abuse and interpersonal violence. As it is mandatory for professionals from health and social care to undertake education (and/or training) in child protection, our view is that this should also be similar for adult protection and for those practitioners who will specialise in work with adults. However, this is not yet the case for any of the professional or vocational training courses, although NVQ level 2 has a module concerning abuse and violence (at the level of basic awareness raising). Although we suggested above that such training should be multi-agency in orientation and that this is indicative of good practice in this area, it is also apparent that inter-professional education at pre- and post qualifying level is far from the norm across the UK and that it will take some time to achieve this aspiration. Therefore in the meantime we hope that the different qualifying courses for professionals who will work with adults will begin to develop and adopt education concerning adult protection as a matter of routine.

SUPERVISION AND SUPPORT

Once students have qualified and obtained work, or staff within organisations have progressed beyond induction-level training, there is an ongoing need for regular and consistent supervision and support. A distinction may be drawn here between professional supervision and supervision in relation to managerial requirements for the purposes of the organisation. Clearly in some situations staff may receive one form of supervision rather than both, which then may not meet their needs for ongoing professional (and personal) development. Unfortunately in a few instances, individuals may not receive either form of supervision and may rather be left to their own devices, although it is hoped that this is a comparatively rare occurrence. It is also hoped that staff will be able to access appropriate professional supervision from colleagues and peers, perhaps via systems of group or co-supervision, where necessary.

The issue of support, as distinct from supervision, of whatever type, is also of note here. In order to remain effective in their work, practitioners require support as well as guidance. If the individual is working with vulnerable adults, they are likely at times to need additional support to help them to deal with situations of abuse, violence and neglect and the complexities that these can encompass. This is particularly likely to be the case if there is little that the practitioner can do to effect change in the situation (perhaps owing to circumstances such as the individual service user refusing suggested interventions or even to acknowledge the situation as abusive). If the practitioner remains involved in the situation in some sort of monitoring or review role, it can be very difficult to remain dispassionate and sufficiently emotionally distanced yet still fully committed to the empowerment of the individual.

Input from an effective manager can be of particular value here to support and sustain the practitioner in their role and task. The management of empathy is also essential in relation to this. For a practitioner to remain empathetic and to be able to build and maintain appropriate relationships with service users is evidently crucial to their performance in overall terms. This may perhaps particularly be the case in relation to the undoubtedly complex and sensitive issues that relate to situations involving adult protection. However, it is also necessary for the manager to be able to assess satisfactorily whether the practitioner retains appropriate levels of sensitivity and empathy with service users. If a manager detects that the practitioner is no longer empathetic and sensitive to the needs of the individuals they work with, then the manager must explore this further with the practitioner. This should be done as a matter of both managerial and professional concern, in order to determine why the situation has arisen and what might be done about it.

Arguably, if a practitioner is not able to really sense, appreciate and share the difficulties (including at times the pain) that the service user experiences then they will not be likely to be able to work effectively with that individual (or those individuals) and alternative arrangements should be made. This is necessary not solely in relation to the practitioner but also the service users who are likely to be affected by the situation. The practitioner may need to be moved to another area of work, where there is less pressure and/or stress, and to receive some assistance and support in terms of both professional and personal needs. Yet the service users concerned are likely to require timely, appropriate and tailored responses from practitioners and services that are sensitive to their particular needs and will ensure that they receive sufficient protection, support and safety planning as necessary.

FINAL COMMENTS

Violence, abuse and neglect of vulnerable adults are amongst the last areas of inter-personal violence to be recognised and dealt with. Indeed, responses to these phenomena have been relatively slow to develop either at the micro (organizational and local) level, addressing the needs of particular individuals, or at the macro societal level, addressing the needs at system and socio-structural levels. This would appear to be largely due to the existence of societal discrimination and marginalisation, which is evident towards adults who have needs for care, and at times, treatment. The 'othering' that vulnerable and disadvantaged individuals experience from the wider society also forms a backdrop and context in which abuse and neglect develop and are maintained. And it is this master state of discrimination and marginalisation that must also be resolved if we are to deal successfully with these forms of violence and to find effective ways of preventing reoccurrence and keeping people safe when they require this level of intervention. One of the key challenges is how to tackle, and ultimately prevent, discrimination and social exclusion effectively at all levels at which they occur. Although steps are being taken to achieve this, there is still a long way to go before this is goal is achieved and we evidently need to make further progress in relation to this aspect of social life for those who are disadvantaged and marginalised.

Moreover, the existence of this master status in turn links to the comparative lack of recognition, until relatively recently, that this form of violence, abuse and exploitation is a social problem in need of attention. There is also an established need for further research and both the development and dissemination of knowledge and understanding about violence, abuse and neglect of vulnerable adults. We are now at a stage when there is recognition, albeit somewhat partial, of the existence of a problem requiring action to resolve it, and initial steps are being taken to address the situation. What we now need is a continued willingness and commitment to pursue the achievement of resolution of abusive and neglectful situations, to assist individuals who are affected by such situations and in addition to work towards prevention and the development of preventative strategies. This is likely to be a lengthy journey, but one that is essential to take in order to tackle this most pernicious of problems. We hope that this book provides another marker along that route.

REFERENCES

Action on Elder Abuse (2002) *Abuse in Care Homes*, London: Action on Elder Abuse.

Action on Elder Abuse (2005) *Hidden Voices: Older People's Experience of Abuse: An Analysis of Calls to the Action on Elder Abuse Helpline*, London: Action on Elder Abuse.

Action on Elder Abuse (2006) *Adult Protection Data Collection and Reporting Requirements*, London: Action on Elder Abuse.

Adcroft, A. and Willis, R. (2005) The (un)intended outcome of public sector performance measurement, *International Journal of Public Sector Management*, 18, 5, 386–400.

ADSS (2005) *Safeguarding Adults: A National Framework of Standards for Good Practice and Outcomes in Adult Protection Work*, London: Association of Directors of Social Services.

ALMA (2004) ALMA, France, *Journal of Adult Protection*, 6, 3, 40–2.

Atkinson, D. (1994) Group-based reminiscence with people with learning difficulties. In J. Bornat (ed.) *Reminiscence Reviewed: Perspectives, Evaluations and Achievements*, Buckingham: Open University Press.

Audit Commission (2005) *Comprehensive Performance Assessment – The Harder Test. Scores and Analysis of Performance in Single Tier and County Councils 2005*, London: Audit Commission.

Balloch, S. and Taylor, M. (2001) Introduction. In S. Balloch and M. Taylor (eds) *Partnership Working and Practice*, Bristol: Policy Press.

BASW (2002) *Code of Ethics*, Birmingham: British Association of Social Workers.

Beaulieu, M. and Leclerc, N. (2006) Ethical and psychosocial issues raised by practice in cases of mistreatment in older adults, *Journal of Gerontological Social Work*, 46, 3–4, 161–86.

Beckett, C. and Maynard, A. (2005) *Values and Ethics in Social Work*, London: Sage.

Bennett, G., Kingston, P. and Penhale, B. (1997) *The Dimensions of Elder Abuse: Perspectives for Practitioners*, Basingstoke: Macmillan.

Beresford, P., Adshead, L. and Croft, S. (2007) *Palliative Care, Social Work & Service Users: Making Life Possible*, London: Jessica Kingsley Publishers.

Berger, P. and Luckmann, T. (1966) *The Social Construction of Reality: A Treatise in the Sociology of Knowledge*, London: Penguin Books.

Bichard, R. (2004) *The Bichard Inquiry Report*, HC653, London: The Stationery Office.

BILD (2004) *Factsheet – What Is a Learning Disability?* Kidderminster: British Institute of Learning Disabilities, www.bild.org.uk, accessed April 2006.

Bradley, G. and Manthorpe, J. (1997) *Dilemmas of Financial Assessment*, Birmingham: Venture Press.

Brady, S. M. (2001) Sterilization of girls and women with intellectual disabilities: past and present justifications, *Violence Against Women*, 7, 4, 432–61.

Brammer, A. (1999) A fit person to run a home: registered homes tribunal interpretations of the 'fit person' concept in the United Kingdom, *Journal of Elder Abuse and Neglect*, 10, 2, 119–31.

Brammer, A. (2006) *Social Work Law* (2nd edition), Harlow: Pearson.

Brayne, H. and Carr, H. (2005) *Law for Social Workers* (9th edition), Oxford: Oxford University Press.

Brogden, M. and Nijhar, P. (2000) *Crime, Abuse and the Elderly*, Cullompton: Willan Publishing.

Brown, H. (1999) Abuse of people with learning disabilities: layers of concern and analysis. In N. Stanley, J. Manthorpe and B. Penhale (eds) *Institutional Abuse: Perspectives across the Life Course*, London: Routledge.

Brown, H. and Stein, J. (1998) Implementing adult protection policies in Kent and East Sussex, *Journal of Social Policy*, 27, 3, 371–96.

Brown, H. and Thompson, D. (1997) Service responses to men with intellectual disabilities who have sexually abusive or unacceptable behaviours: the case against inaction, *Journal of Applied Research in Intellectual Disability*, 10, 2, 176–97. `

Brown, H., Stein, J. and Turk, V. (1995) The sexual abuse of adults with learning disabilities: report of a second two year incidence survey, *Mental Handicap Research*, 8, 1, 3–24.

Brownell, P. (1997) The application of the culturagram in cross-cultural practice with elder abuse victims, *Journal of Elder Abuse and Neglect*, 9, 2, 19–33.

Busby, F. (2004) ALMA, France, *Journal of Adult Protection*, 6, 3, 45–6.

Butler, S. and Lymbery, M. (2004) *Social Work Ideals and Practice Realities*, Basingstoke: Macmillan.

Callahan, J. (1988) Elder abuse: some questions for policymakers, *Gerontologist*, 28, 4, 453–8.

Cambridge, P., Beadle-Brown, J., Milne, A., Mansell, J. and Whelton, B. (2006) *Analysis of Adult Protection Referrals*, press release, Canterbury: Tizard Centre, University of Kent.

Casasola, A. (2005) *Telefono anziani maltrattati: presentati i dati del 2004*, Udine: Provincia di Udine.

Casey, C., Hazlett, S.-A. and McAdam, R. (2005) Performance management in the UK public sector: addressing multiple stakeholder complexity, *International Journal of Public Sector Management*, 18, 3, 256–73.

Castles, S. and Miller, M. J. (1998) *The Age of Migration: International Population Movements in the Modern World*, Basingstoke: Macmillan.

Cemlyn, S. and Briskman, L. (2003) Asylum, children's rights and social work, *Child and Family Social Work*, 8, 163–78.

Chang, J., Martin, S., Moracco, K., Dulli, L., Scandlin, D., Louckes-Sorrel, M., Turner, T., Starsonek, L., Dorian, P. and Bou-Saada, I. (2003) Helping women with disabilities and domestic violence: strategies, limitations and challenges of domestic violence programs and services, *Journal of Women's Health*, 12, 7, 699–708.

Civjan, S. (2000) Making sexual assault and domestic violence services accessible, *Impact: Feature Issue on Violence Against Women with Developmental or Other Disabilites*, 13, 3, http://www.ici.umn.edu/products/newsletters, accessed 16 December 2006.

Clarke, J. and Glendinning, C. (2003) Partnerships and the remaking of welfare governance. In C. Glendinning, M. Powell and K. Rummery (eds) *Partnerships, New Labour and the Governance of Welfare*, Bristol: Policy Press.

Clough, R. (1994) *Insights into Inspection: The Regulation of Social Care*, London: Whiting and Birch.

Clough, R. (1996) *Abuse of Care in Residential Institutions*, London: Whiting and Birch.

Clough, R. (1999) Scandalous care: interpreting public inquiry reports of scandals in residential care, *Journal of Elder Abuse and Neglect*, 10, 1/2, 13–27.

Cochrane, R. (1983) *The Social Creation of Mental Illness*, London: Longman.

Collins, P. (2005) *Values and Mental Capacity*, London: Mental Health Foundation.

Colmo, G. (2006) Roma: anziani nel mirino dei ladri. Agenzia d'informazione, *AUSER*, 9, 40.

Commission for Health Improvement (2003) *Investigation into Matters Arising from Care on Rowan Ward, Manchester Mental Health and Social Care Trust*, London: The Stationery Office.

Commission for Healthcare Audit and Inspection (2006) *State of Healthcare 2006*, London: The Stationery Office.

Congress, E. (1994) The use of culturagrams to assess and empower culturally diverse families, *Families in Society*, 75, 9, 531–40.

Copperman, J. and McNamara, J. (1999) Institutional abuse in mental health settings: survivor perspectives. In N. Stanley, J. Manthorpe and B. Penhale (eds) *Institutional Abuse: Perspectives across the Life Course*, London: Routledge, pp. 152–72.

Coulshed, V. and Orme, J. (2006) *Social Work Practice: An Introduction* (4th edition), Basingstoke: Palgrave.

Coulshed, V., Mullender, A. with Jones, D. and Thompson, N. (2006) *Management in Social Work* (3rd edition), Basingstoke: Palgrave.

Counsel & Care (1995) *In Harm's Way*, London: Counsel & Care.

Cozens, A. (2006) Use your imagination, *Community Care*, 19–25 October, 38–40.

CSCI (2005a) *Social Services Performance Assessment Framework Indicators 2004–2005*, London: Commission for Social Care Inspection.

CSCI (2005b) *Inspecting for Better Lives – Delivering Change*, London: Commission for Social Care Inspection.

CSCI (2005c) *Social Care Performance, 20-04-05*, Newcastle: Commission for Social Care Inspection.

CSCI (2006) *Care Homes Fail on Medication Standards*, London: Commission for Social Care Inspection.

CSCI and Healthcare Commission (2006) *Joint Investigation into the Provision of Services for People with Learning Disabilities at Cornwall Partnership NHS Trust*, Commission for Healthcare Audit and Inspection, http://www.healthcarecomission.org.uk/_db/_documents/cornwall_investigation_report.pdf, accessed August 2006.

CSIP (2005) *The Social Work Contribution to Mental Health Services: The Future Direction. A Discussion Paper*, London: CSIP.

Dalrymple, J. and Burke, B. (1995) *Anti-oppressive Practice: Social Care and the Law*, Buckingham: Open University Press.

Dean, R., Proudfoot, R. and Lindesay, J. (1993) The Quality of Interactions Schedule (QUIS): development, reliability and use in the evaluation of two domus units, *International Journal of Geriatric Psychiatry*, 8, 819–26.

Department for Constitutional Affairs (2003) *Public Sector Data Sharing: Guidance on the Law*, London: Department for Constitutional Affairs.

Department for Constitutional Affairs (2007) *Mental Capacity Act 2005 Code of Practice (2007 Final Edition)*, London: The Stationery Office.

Department of Health (1989) *Caring for People: Community Care in the Next Decade and Beyond*, Cmnd 849, London: HMSO.

Department of Health (1995) *Elder Abuse: Report of Two National Seminars*, London: Department of Health.

Department of Health (1998a) *Partnerships in Action: New Opportunities for Joint Working between Health and Social Services*, London: Department of Health.

Department of Health (1998b) *Modernising Social Services*, London: Department of Health.

Department of Health (1998c) *Modernising Mental Health Services*, London: The Stationery Office.

Department of Health (1999a) *National Service Framework for Mental Health*, London: The Stationery Office.

Department of Health (1999b) *Protecting and Using Patient Information: A Manual for Caldicott Guardians*, London: The Stationery Office.

Department of Health (2000a) *No Secrets: Guidance on Developing and Implementing Multi-agency Policies and Procedures to Protect Vulnerable Adults from Abuse*, London: Department of Health.

Department of Health (2000b) *The National Health Plan*, London: The Stationery Office.

Department of Health (2000c) *Reforming the Mental Health Act*, Cmnd 5016-I-II, London: The Stationery Office.

Department of Health (2001a) *Valuing People: A New Strategy for Learning Disability for the 21st Century*, London: Department of Health.

Department of Health (2001b) *National Service Framework for Older People*, London: The Stationery Office.

Department of Health (2002a) *Learning Disabilities: Facts and Figures*, http://www.dh.gov. uk/PolicyAndGuidance/HealthAndSocialCareTopics/Learningdisabilities, accessed June 2006.

Department of Health (2002b) *Implementing the Caldicott Standard into Social Care HSC 2002–2003: LCA (2002)2*, London: Department of Health.

Department of Health (2003a) *Fair Access to Care Services: Guidance on Eligibility Criteria for Adult Social Care*, London: Department of Health.

Department of Health (2003b) *Delivering Race Equality: A Framework for Action*, London: The Stationery Office.

Department of Health (2004) *Protection of Vulnerable Adults in England and Wales for Care Homes and Domiciliary Care Agencies*, London: Department of Health.

Department of Health (2005a) *Independence, Well-being and Choice*, London: Department of Health.

Department of Health (2005b) *Mental Capacity Act 2005*, London: The Stationery Office.

Department of Health (2005c) *The National Service Framework for Long Term Conditions*, London: Department of Health.

Department of Health (2006a) *Our Health, Our Care, Our Say: A New Direction for Community Services*, London: Department of Health.

Department of Health (2006b) *Mental Health Bill*, London: Department of Health.

Department of Health (2006c) *The Expert Patient: A New Approach to Chronic Disease Management for the 21st Century*, London: Department of Health.

Department of Health (2007) *A Recipe for Care: Not a Single Ingredient*, London: Department of Health.

DHSS (1969) *Report of the Committee of Inquiry into Allegations of Ill-treatment and Other Irregularities at Ely Hospital, Cardiff*, Cmnd 3785, London: HMSO.

DHSS (1971a) *Better Services for the Mentally Handicapped*, Cmnd 4683, London: HMSO.

DHSS (1971b) *Report of the Farleigh Hospital Committee of Inquiry*, Cmnd 4557, London: HMSO.

DHSS (1972) *Report of the Committee of Inquiry into Whittingham Hospital*, Cmnd 4871, London: HMSO.

Disability Services ASAP (2000) *Stop the Violence, Break the Silence – Resource Kit*, Austin, TX: Austin Safe-Place.

Doel, M. and Shardlow, S. M. (2005) *Modern Social Work Practice: Teaching and Learning in Practice Settings*, Aldershot: Ashgate.

Dominelli, L. (1997) *Anti-racist Social Work* (2nd edition), Basingstoke: Macmillan.

Dominelli, L. (2002) *Anti-oppressive Social Work Theory and Practice*, Basingstoke: Palgrave.

Eastman, M. (1984) At worst just picking up the pieces, *Community Care*, 2 February, 20–2.

Eaton, W. (1980) *The Sociology of Mental Disorders*, New York: Praeger.

Edwards, M. and Miller, C. (2003) *Integrating Health and Social Care and Making it Work*, London: Office of Public Management.

Emerson, E., Hatton, C., Felce, D. and Murphy, G. (2001) *Learning Disabilities: The Fundamental Facts*, London: Foundation for People with Learning Disabilities.

Emerson, E., Malam, B., Davies, I. and Spencer, K. (2005) *A Survey of Adults with a Learning Disability in 2003–04*, National Statistics and NHS Health and Social Care Information, www.dh.gov.uk/PublicationsAndStatistics/PublishedSurvey/ListofSurveyssince1990/GeneralSurveys/GeneralSurveysArticle/fs/en?/CONTENT_ID=4081207&chk=u%Bdsfvv, accessed July 2006.

Fairfax, P., Green, E. and South, J. (2005) Developing an assessment tool for evaluating community involvement, *Health Expectations*, 8, 1, 64–73.

Fletcher, K. (2006) *Partnerships in Social Care*, London: Jessica Kingsley.

Flynn, M. (2006) Viewpoint, *Journal of Adult Protection*, 8, 3, 28–32.

Friedman, M. and Friedman, R. (1962) *Capitalism and Freedom*, Chicago: University of Chicago Press.

Frohmader, C. (1998) *Violence against Women with Disabilities – a Report from the National Women with Disabilities and Violence Workshop*, Melbourne: Women with Disabilities, Australia.

Galtung, J. and Tord, H. (1971) Structural and direct violence: a note on operationalisation, *Journal of Peace Research*, 8, 73–6.

Garrett, P. M. (2002) 'No Irish need apply': social work and the history and politics of exclusionary paradigms and practices, *British Journal of Social Work*, 32, 4, 477–94.

Gates, B. (ed.) (2003) *Learning Disabilities: Towards Inclusion* (4th edition), London: Churchill Livingstone.

Gibson, F. (2004) *The Past in the Present: Using Reminiscence in Health and Social Care*, Baltimore, MD: Health Professions Press.

Giddens, A. (1998) *The Third Way: The Renewal of Social Democracy*, Cambridge: Polity Press.

Goergen, T. (2006) Elder abuse prevention strategies in Germany, Paper given at conference on Violence and Grave Neglect of the Elderly, Cologne.

Goffman, E. (1961) *Asylums*, New York: Doubleday.

Goldthorpe, L. (2004) Every child matters: a legal perspective, *Child Abuse Review*, 13, 115–36.

Golightley, M. (2006) *Social Work and Mental Health* (2nd edition), Exeter: Learning Matters.

GSCC (2002) *Codes of Practice for Employees and Employers*, London: General Social Care Council.

Gunn, J. (2000) Future directions for treatment in forensic psychiatry, *British Journal of Psychiatry*, 176, 332–8.

Ham, C. (2006) Creative destruction in the NHS, *British Medical Journal*, 332, 7548, 984–5.

Harris, J. (2004) Consumerism: social development or social delimitation, *International Social Work*, 47, 4, 533–42.

Hayes, D. (2005) Social work with asylum seekers and others subject to immigration control. In R. Adams, L. Dominelli and M. Payne (eds) *Social Work Futures: Crossing Boundaries, Transforming Practice*, Basingstoke: Palgrave.

Hayes, D. and Humphries, B. (2004) *Social Work, Immigration and Asylum*, London: Jessica Kingsley Publishers.

Healthcare Commission (2006) *Joint Investigation into the Provision of Services for People with Learning Disabilities at Cornwall Partnership NHS Trust*, London: Commission for Healthcare Audit and Inspection.

Healthcare Commission (2007) *Investigation into the Service for People with Learning Disabilities Provided by Sutton and Merton Primary Care Trust*, London: Commission for Healthcare Audit and Inspection.

Hightower, J. and Smith, M. (2002) *Silent and Invisibile: What's Age Got to Do with It? A Handbook for Service Providers on Working with Abused Older Women in British Columbia and Yukon*, Vancouver, BC: Yukon Society of Transition Houses.

Hightower, J., Hightower, H. and Smith, M. (2006) Hearing the voices of abused older women, *Journal of Gerontological Social Work*, 46, 3–4, 205–27.

Hightower, J., Smith, M., Ward-Hall, C. and Hightower, H. (1999) Meeting the needs of abused older women, *Journal of Elder Abuse and Neglect*, 11, 4, 39–58.

Home Office (2001) *Action for Justice*, London: Home Office.

Home Office (2003) *Achieving Best Evidence in Criminal Proceedings: Guidance for Vulnerable and Intimidated Witnesses, Including Children. Consultation Draft*. London: Home Office.

Horner, N. (2006) *What Is Social Work? Context and Perspectives* (2nd edition), Exeter: Learning Matters.

Howe, D. (1998) Relationship-based thinking and practice in social work, *Journal of Social Work Practice*, 12, 45–56.

Hubert, J. and Hollins, S. (2006) Men with severe learning disabilities and challenging behaviour in long-stay hospital care, *British Journal of Psychiatry*, 188, 1, 70–4.

Hudson, B. and Hardy, B. (2002) What is successful partnership and how can it be measured? In C. Glendinning, M. Powell and K. Rummery (eds) *Partnerships, New Labour and the Governance of Welfare*, Bristol: Policy Press.

Hugman, R. (2005) *New Approaches in Ethics for the Caring Professions*, Basingstoke: Palgrave.

Hydle, I. and Johns, S. (1992) *Stengte dører og knyttede never: når eldre blir utsatt for overgrep i hjemmet*, Oslo: Kommuneforlaget.

Jack, R. (1994) Dependence, power and violation: gender issues in the abuse of elderly people by formal carers. In M. Eastman (ed.) *Old Age Abuse*, London: Chapman & Hall.

Jack, R. (1998) (ed.) *Residential Versus Community Care*, Basingstoke: Macmillan.

Jackson, C. (2006) Out of sight, *Mental Health Today*, September, 8–9.

Johns, R. (2005) *Using the Law in Social Work Practice*, Exeter: Learning Matters.

Johns, R. (2007) *Using the Law in Social Work* (3rd edition), Exeter: Learning Matters.

Johns, R. and Sedgwick, A. (1998) *Law for Social Work Practice: Work with Vulnerable Adults*, Basingstoke: Macmillan.

Johns, S. and Juklestad, O. (1995) *Vern for eldre: prosjektrapport. Universitetsseksjonen, geriatrisk avdeling*, Oslo: Ullevål Sykehus.

Johnson, M. (2006) Report review: National Patient Safety Report, *Journal of Adult Protection*, 8, 3, 36–8.

Jordan, B. (2000) *Social Work and the Third Way: Tough Love as Social Policy*, London: Sage.

Juklestad, O. (2001) Institutional care: the dark side, *Journal of Adult Protection*, 3, 2, 32–41.

Jukelstad, O. (2004) Elderly people at risk: a Norwegian model for community education and response, *Journal of Adult Protection*, 6, 3, 26–33.

Keating, F. and Robertson, D. (2004) Fear, black people and mental illness: a vicious circle?, *Health and Social Care in the Community*, 12, 5, 439–47.

Kelly, B. (2005) Structural violence and schizophrenia, *Social Science and Medicine*, 61, 721–30.

Khan, P. (2003) An analysis of conflict experienced between agencies involved with asylum seekers, *Journal of Social Work Practice*, 17, 1, 115–26.

Kidane, S. (2001a) *Food, Shelter and Half a Chance: Assessing the Needs of Unaccompanied Asylum Seeking Children*, London: British Association for Adoption and Fostering.

Kidane, S. (2001b) *I Did Not Choose to Come Here: Listening to Refugee Children*, London: British Association for Adoption and Fostering.

Kitchen, S. and Elliott, R. (2001) *Key Findings from the Vulnerable Witness Survey*, Findings 147, London: Home Office.

Kitwood, T. (1997) *Dementia Reconsidered: The Person Comes First*, Buckingham: Open University Press.

Kumar, K. (1978) *Prophecy and Progress*. Harmondsworth: Penguin Books.

Laing, R. and Esterson, A. (1970) *Sanity, Madness and the Family*, London: Pelican.

Lavalette, M., Ferguson, I. and Mooney, G. (2002) *Rethinking Welfare: A Critical Perspective*, London: Sage.

Lefley, H. (1987) Aging parents as caregivers of mentally ill adult children: an emerging social problem, *Hospital and Community Psychiatry*, 38, 1063–70.

Lefley, H. (1996) *Family Caregiving in Mental Illness*, Thousand Oaks, CA: Sage.

Lindesay, J., Briggs, K., Lawes, M., Macdonald, A. and Herzberg, J. (1991) The Domus philosophy: a comparative evaluation of a new approach to residential care for the demented elderly, *International Journal of Geriatric Psychiatry*, 6, 727–36.

Lord Chancellor's Department (1998) *Who Decides? Making Decisions on Behalf of Mentally Incapacitated Adults*, London: The Stationery Office.

Lord Chancellor's Department (2007) *Mental Capacity Act 2005: Code of Practice*, London: The Stationery Office.

Loxley, A. (1997) *Collaboration in Health and Welfare: Working with Difference*, London: Jessica Kingsley.

Mac an Ghaill, M. (2000) The Irish in Britain: the invisibility of ethnicity and anti-Irish racism, *Journal of Ethnic and Migration Studies*, 26, 1, 137–47.

McCarthy, M. (2000) An evaluation research study of a specialist women's refuge, *Journal of Adult Protection*, 2, 2, 29–40.

McDonald, A. (1999) *Understanding Community Care*, Basingstoke: Macmillan.

McDonald, P. and Coleman, M. (1999) Deconstructing hierarchies of oppression and adopting a 'multiple model' approach to anti-oppressive practice, *Social Work Education*, 18, 1, 19–33.

Macpherson Report (1999) *The Stephen Lawrence Inquiry: Report of an Inquiry by Sir William Macpherson of Cluny*, London: The Stationery Office.

Maes, B. and Van Puyenbroeck, J. (2005) Reminiscence in ageing people with intellectual disabilities: an exploratory study, *British Journal of Developmental Disabilities*, 51, 1, 3–16.

Mandelstam, M. (1999) *Community Care Practice and the Law* (2nd edition), London: Jessica Kingsley.

Manthorpe, J. (1999) Users' perceptions: searching for the views of users with learning disabilities. In N. Stanley, J. Manthorpe and B. Penhale (eds) *Institutional Abuse: Perspectives across the Life Course*, London: Routledge.

Marshall, J. (2006) Performance management: causes and effects and their impact on community care. In K Brown (ed.) *Vulnerable Adults and Community Care*, Exeter: Learning Matters.

Marsland, D., Oakes, P., Tweddell, I. and White, C. (2006) *Abuse in Care? A Practical Guide to Protecting People with Learning Disabilities from Abuse in Residential Services*, Hull: Faculty of Health and Social Care, University of Hull.

Mason, D. (1995) *Race and Ethnicity in Modern Britain*, Oxford: Oxford University Press.

Mayo, M. (2002) Community work. In R. Adams, L. Dominelli and M. Payne (eds) *Social Work: Themes, Issues and Critical Debates* (2nd edition), Basingstoke: Palgrave.

Mears, J. and Sargent, M. (2002) *More than Survival: Project Report Two for Professionals*. Sydney: University of Western Sydney.

Mental Health Act Commission (2005) *In Place of Fear? 11th Biennial Report 2003–2005*, London: Mental Health Act Commission.

Mental Health Act Commission / Sainsbury Centre for Mental Health (2000) *The National One Day Visit*, London: Mental Health Act Commission.

METIS project (1998) *Guide on Violence and Disabled Women*, Brussels: DAPHNE programme, EU Commission.

Milner, J. and O'Byrne, P. (2002) *Assessment in Social Work* (2nd edition), Basingstoke: Palgrave.

Ministry of Health (1962) *A Hospital Plan for England and Wales*, Cmnd 1604, London: HMSO.

Moriarty, J. and Levin, E. (1998) Respite care in homes and hospitals. In R. Jack (ed.) *Residential Versus Community Care*, Basingstoke: Macmillan.

Murphy, G. and Clare, I. (1995) Adults' capacity to make decisions affecting the person: psychologists' contribution. In R. Bull and D. Carson (eds) *Handbook of Psychology in Legal Contexts*, Chichester: Wiley.

National Assembly for Wales (2000) *In Safe hands: Implementing Adult Protection in Wales*, Cardiff: National Assembly for Wales. Available from: http://www.wales.gov.uk/subisocialpolicy/content/pdf/safehands_e.pdf, accessed 10 January 2004.

National Audit Office (2005) *A Safer Place for Patients: Learning to Improve Patient Safety*, HC 456, Parliamentary Session 2005–6, London: National Audit Office.

National Patient Safety Agency and the Patient Safety Observatory (2006) *With Safety in Mind: Mental Health Services and Patient Safety*, London: National Patient Safety Agency.

Nazroo, J. (1999) *Ethnicity and Mental Health*, London: Policy Studies Institute.

Newton, J. (1988) *Preventing Mental Illness*, London: Routledge.

Nomme Russell, M. and White, B. (2002) Social worker and immigrant client experiences in multicultural service provision: educational implications, *Social Work Education*, 21, 6, 635–50.

O'Callaghan, A. C., Murphy, G. and Clare, I. C. H. (2003) The impact of abuse on men and women with severe learning disabilities and their families, *British Journal of Learning Disabilities*, 31, 175–80.

Office of the Deputy Prime Minister (ODPM) (2004) *Mental Health and Social Exclusion, Social Exclusion Unit Report*, London: The Stationery Office.

Oliver, M. (1983) *Social Work with Disabled People*, Basingstoke: Macmillan.

Oliver, M. (1990) *The Politics of Disablement*, Basingstoke: Macmillan.

Panayi, P. (1999) *The Impact of Immigration: A Documentary History of the Effects and Experiences of Immigrants in Britain since 1945*, Manchester: Manchester University Press.

Parker, J. (1998) The prevention and management of elder abuse. In K. Cigno and D. Bourn (eds) *Cognitive-behavioural Social Work in Practice*, Aldershot: Arena/Ashgate.

Parker, J. (2000) Social work with refugees and asylum seekers: a rationale for developing practice, *Practice*, 12, 3, 61–76.

Parker, J. (2007a) The process of social work: assessment, planning, intervention and review. In M. Lymbery and K. Postle (eds) *Social Work: A Companion to Learning*, London: Sage.

Parker, J. (2007b) Social work, disadvantage by association and anti-oppressive practice. In P. Burke and J. Parker (eds) *Social Work and Disadvantage: Addressing the Roots of Stigma through Association*, London: Jessica Kingsley.

Parker, J. and Bradley, G. (2003) *Social Work Practice: Assessment, Planning, Intervention and Review*, Exeter: Learning Matters.

Payne, M. (1995) *Social Work and Community Care*, Basingstoke: Macmillan.

Payne, M. (2005) *The Origins of Social Work: Continuity and Change*, Basingstoke: Palgrave.

Peace, S. and Holland, C. (1998) *Homely Residential Care: The Report of a Pilot Study of Small Homes for Older People Carried out in Bedfordshire*, Buckingham: Open University Press.

Peace, S., Kellaher, L. and Willcocks, D. (1997) *Re-evaluating Residential Care*, Buckingham: Open University Press.

Penhale, B. (1999) Introduction. In N. Stanley, J. Manthorpe and B. Penhale (eds) *Institutional Abuse: Perspectives across the Life Course*, London: Routledge.

Penhale, B. and Manthorpe, J. (2004) Older people, institutional abuse and inquiries. In N. Stanley and J. Manthorpe (eds) *The Age of the Inquiry: Learning and Blaming in Health and Social Care*, London: Routledge.

Penhale, B. and Parker, J. with Kingston, P. (2000) *Elder Abuse*, Birmingham: Venture Press.

Penhale, B., Perkins, N., Pinkney, L., Reid, D., Manthorpe, J. and Hussein, S. (2007) *Partnerships and Regulation in Adult Protection: Final Report to the Department of Health*, London: Department of Health.

Penrose, L. (1939) Mental disease and crime: outline of a comparative study of European statistics, *British Journal of Medical Psychology*, 18, 1–15.

Perkins, N., Penhale, B., Pinkney, L., Reid, D., Manthorpe, J. and Hussein, S. (2007) Partnership means protection? The effectiveness of multi-agency working and the regulatory framework in adult protection, *Journal of Adult Protection*, 9, 3, 9–23.

Perring, C. (1992) The experience and perspectives of patients and care staff of the transition from hospital to community based care. In S. Ramon (ed.) *Psychiatric Hospital Closure: Myths and Realities*, London: Chapman & Hall.

Phillipson, C. and Biggs, S. (1995) Elder abuse: a critical overview. In P. Kingston and B. Penhale (eds) *Family Violence and the Caring Professions*, Basingstoke: Macmillan.

Popple, K. (1995) *Analysing Community Work: Its Theory and Practice*, Buckingham: Open University Press.

Postle, K. (2002) Working 'between the idea and the reality' – ambiguities and tensions in care managers' work, *British Journal of Social Work*, 32, 3, 335–51.

Prairie Rose (1995) Elder abuse: what it is and how the Senior Line can help, *Prairie Rose*, 64, 2, 19–20.

Pritchard, C. (2006) *Mental Health Social Work: Evidence-based Practice*, London: Routledge.

Pritchard, J. (2000) *The Needs of Older Women*, Bristol: Policy Press.

Pritchard, J. (2003) *Support Groups for Older People who Have Been Abused: Beyond Existing*, London: Jessica Kingsley.

Proctor, E. K. (2002) Quality of care and social work research, *Social Work Research*, 26, 4, 195–7.

Quinney, A. (2006) *Collaborative Social Work Practice*, Exeter: Learning Matters.

Randall, P. (1997) *Adult Bullying: Perpetrators and Victims*, London: Routledge.

Reingold, D. (2006) An elder abuse shelter program: build it and they will come, a long-term care based program to address elder abuse in the community, *Journal of Gerontological Social Work*, 46, 3–4, 125–35.

Richardson, S. and Asthana, S. (2005) Policy and legal influences on inter-organisational information sharing in health and social care services, *Journal of Integrated Care*, 13, 3, 3–10.

Roberto, K., Teaster, P. and Duke, J. (2004) Older women who experience mistreatment: circumstances and outcomes, *Journal of Women and Aging*, 16, 2, 3–16.

Royal College of Psychiatrists' Research Unit (2005) *The National Audit of Violence 2003–2005 Final Report*, London: Royal College of Psychiatrists.

Rutter, J. (2001) *Supporting Refugee Children in 21st Century Britain: A Compendium of Essential Information*, Stoke: Trentham Books.

Sainsbury Centre for Mental Health (1997) *The National Visit: A One-day Visit to 309 Acute Psychiatric Wards by the Mental Health Act Commission in Collaboration with The Sainsbury Centre for Mental Health*, London: The Sainsbury Centre for Mental Health.

Sargent, M. and Mears, J. (2002) *More than Survival: Project Report One for Older Women*, Sydney: University of Western Sydney.

Sayce, L. (2003) *Mental Health and Citizenship*, London: Mind Books.

Schaffer, J. (1999) Older and isolated women and domestic violence project, *Journal of Elder Abuse and Neglect*, 11, 1, 59–73.

Scull, A. (1979) *Museums of Madness*, London: Allen Lane.

Smale, G., Tucson, G. and Statham, D. (2000) *Social Work and Social Problems*, Basingstoke: Macmillan.

Smith, J. (2002) Department of Health press release. Ref. 2002/0241, http://www.Info.doh.gov.uk/intpress.nsf/page/2002-024111/OpenDocument, accessed 20 October 2002.

Smith, K. and Tilney, S. (2007) *Vulnerable Adult and Child Witnesses*, Oxford: Blackstone.

Sobsey, D. (2000) Faces of violence against women with disabilities, *Impact: Feature Issue on Violence Against Women with Developmental or Other Disabilities*, 13, 3, http://www. ici.umn.edu/products/newsletters, accessed 15 December 2006.

Social Trends (2002) *Social Trends, 1999–2001*, London: OPCS.

Solomos, J. and Beck, L. (1996) *Racism and Society*, Basingstoke: Macmillan.

Stanko, B., O'Beirne, M. and Zaffuto, G. (2002) *Taking Stock: What Do We Know about Interpersonal Violence?* London: ESRC/Royal Holloway.

Stanley N. and Flynn, M. (2005) Editorial, *Journal of Adult Protection*, 7, 4, 1–3.

Stanley, N., Manthorpe, J. and Penhale, B. (eds) (1999) *Institutional Abuse: Perspectives across the Life Course*, London: Routledge.

Steinmetz, S. (1990) Elder abuse: myth and reality. In T. H. Brubaker (ed.) *Family Relationships in Later Life* (2nd edition), Newbury Park, CA: Sage.

Strong and Prosperous Communites. Available from http://www.communities.gov.uk, accessed 3 November 2006.

Sullivan, M. (1996) *The Development of the British Welfare State*, Hemel Hempstead: Prentice Hall/Harvester Wheatsheaf.

Supporting Police, Protecting Communities (2005) http://www.scotland.gov.uk/Publications/ 2005/06/0394432/44339, accessed August 2006.

Szasz, T. (1972) *The Myth of Mental Illness*, London: Paladin.

Talbot, C. (2001) UK public services and management (1979–2000): evolution or revolution? *International Journal of Public Sector Management*, 14, 4, 281–303.

Teaster, P. and Roberto, K. (2004) Sexual abuse of older adults: APS cases and outcomes, *The Gerontologist*, 44, 6, 788–96.

Tett, L. (2006) *Community Education: Lifelong Learning and Social Inclusion*, Edinburgh: Dunedin Academic Press.

Tew, J. (2002) Going social: championing a holistic model of mental distress within professional education, *Social Work Education*, 21, 2, 143–55.

Thomas, M. and Pierson, J. (2006) *Collins Dictionary of Social Work* (2nd edition), London: Collins.

Thompson, N. (2006) *Anti Discriminatory Practice* (4th edition), Basingstoke: Palgrave.

Torode, R., Walsh, T. and Woods, M. with Galvin, T. and Keogh, A. (2001) *Working with Refugees and Asylum Seekers: A Social Work Resource Book*, Dublin: Department of Social Studies, Trinity College.

Tsui, M. (2005) *Social Work Supervision: Contexts and Concepts*, London: Sage.

Turk, V. and Brown, H. (1993) The sexual abuse of adults with learning disabilities: results of a two-year incidence survey, *Mental Handicap Research*, 6, 193–216.

Walmsley, J. and Rolph, S. (2002) The history of community care for people with learning difficulties. In B. Bytheway, V. Bacigalupo, J. Bornat, J. Johnson and S. Spurr (eds) *Understanding Care, Welfare and Community: A Reader*, London: Routledge.

Wardhaugh, J. and Wilding, P. (1993) Towards an explanation of the corruption of care, *Critical Social Policy*, 13, 1, 4–31.

Warren, J. (2007) *Social Work and Service Users*, Exeter: Learning Matters.

Weaver, H. N. and Burns, B. J. (2001) 'I shout with fear at night': understanding the traumatic experiences of refugees and asylum seekers, *Journal of Social Work*, 1, 2, 147–64.

Webb, S. A. (2006) *Social Work in a Risk Society: Social and Political Perspectives*, Basingstoke: Palgrave.

WHO (2001) *World Health Report*, Geneva: World Health Organisation.

Willetts, C., Essex, M., Philpott, A., Zsigo, S. and Assey, J. (2006) Eclectic models in working with learning disabled people – an overview of some key issues concerning health and wellness. In K. Brown (ed.) *Vulnerable Adults and Community Care*, Exeter: Learning Matters.

Williams, J. (2002) Public law protection of vulnerable adults: the debate continues, so does the abuse, *Journal of Social Work*, 2, 3, 293–316.

Williams, J. and Keating, F. (1999) The abuse of adults in mental health settings. In N. Stanley, J. Manthorpe and B. Penhale (eds) *Institutional Abuse: Perspectives across the Life Course*, London: Routledge, pp. 130–51.

Williams, J. and Keating, F. (2000) Abuse in mental health services: some theoretical considerations, *Journal of Adult Protection*, 2, 3, 17.

Williams, P. (2006) *Social Work with People with Learning Difficulties*, Exeter: Learning Matters.

Wisseman, K. (2000) 'You're my pretty bird in a cage': disability, domestic violence and survival, *Impact: Feature Issue on Violence Against Women with Developmental or Other Disabilities*, 13, 3, http://www.ici.umn.edu/products/newsletters, accessed 15 December 2006.

Wolff, N. (2005) Community reintegration of prisoners with mental illness: a social investment perspective, *International Journal of Law and Psychiatry*, 28, 43–58.

Women with Disabilities Australia (1999) National Project on Violence Against Women with Disabilities, *Women with Disabilities Australia News*, 16.

Wood, E. (2006) The availability and utility of inter-disciplinary data on elder abuse: a White Paper for the National Center on Elder Abuse, Washington: National Center on Elder Abuse, http://www.elderabusecenter.org, accessed 15 January 2007.

INDEX

Note: Page references in bold refer to figures or tables

abuse: assessment of 72–7; in care settings
  29–35, **31**, **32**, 52, **80–1**; by carers 75–6,
  142–5; community-level 149–64; court
  cases 122, 125, 128–9; criminality of 30,
  32–3, 38, 125, 126; defining 24–7, 29;
  directions of abuse in care settings 30, **31**;
  failure of duty of care 17; helplines 147;
  homophobic 152; individuals' abilities to
  cope with 167; institutional 27–35, **32**;
  interventions in 51–2, **80–1**, 114–15, **115**,
  125–8, 146–8, 166–8; learning disabilities
  and 121–5; levels of abuse 30–1, 80, **80–1**;
  long-term health conditions and 141–5,
  148; mental health difficulties and
  110–15, **115**; power and 12, 14; racist 28,
  29; by relatives 81; social construction of
  25–6; structural 29; support groups for
  victims of 168; systemic 29–30;
  transphobic 152; types of 27–33; welfare
  argument of 30, 32, 38, 125; *see also*
  discriminatory abuse; domestic abuse;
  sexual abuse
accountability 9, **56**
Achieving Best Evidence 88
Action for Justice 88
Action on Elder Abuse 83, 94, 142, 147
acts of omission 28
Adult Protection Committees (APCs) 89–90,
  94
adult protection procedures: education in
  169; guidance on 68–71; inter-agency
  collaboration 87–94; investigations
  69–71, 83–4; levels of engagement in 158;
  for people with learning disabilities 122,
  125; for people with mental health
problems 110, 112, 113; for people with
  physical health difficulties 142;
  prioritising 91; standards on adult
  protection (ADSS) 50; statutory mandate
  for 89; training in 12, 62–3, 84, 122–3,
  169; in the United States 167
Adult Support and Protection Act (Scotland)
  38–9
aids to daily living 133–4
ALMA (Allo Maltraitance des Personnes
  Agées) 147
anger management 77
anti-bullying policies 128
anti-discriminatory practice versus
  anti-oppressive practice 153–4
anti-harassment policies 81, 128
anti-oppressive practice 153–8; versus
  anti-discriminatory practice 153–4; case
  studies 162–3; models of 155–8; working
  with asylum seekers and 160
assessment 65–78; abuse and 72–7; care
  plans 9, 66, 70–1, 75–6, 85–6, 135; case
  conferences 69, 70–1; Community Care
  Assessments 8, 9, 18, 66; continuous 71;
  guidance on protection policies and
  procedures 68–71; information gathering
  and 84–7, **85**, 126–7; interlocking
  patterns of **85**; interviews 73–5, 126–7;
  involving the vulnerable adult 65–6, 70,
  73–4; key elements of the process 67; of
  local authority services 58–60; models of
  social care 67–8; needs-led 66–7; of people
  with learning disabilities 126–7; of people
  with long-term health conditions 138; of
  people with mental health difficulties

114–15, **115**; rights of the vulnerable adult 71–2; risk 73–5, 85; Single Assessment Process 88–9; skills for 69, 76–7; Strategy Meetings 69–70; timing of referrals for 67

Association for Directors of Social Services (ADSS) 50

asylum seekers 158–64

Asylums 102

Audit Commission 58, 59, 61

Australia 127, 147, 148

barring systems 46–8

Beck Depression Inventory 100, 151

Belgium 147

Bennett, G. **80–1**, 168

Best Value Reviews 58, 59

Better Services for the Mentally Handicapped 118, 120

Bexley Community Safety Partnership 152

Bichard Inquiry (2004) 47, 48

bio-psycho-social model 104–6

biological factors for mental health problems 104

Bradford Health Action Zone 61–2

Bradley, G. 65, 71, 76, 123, 163, **164**

Brammer, A. 51

British Association of Social Workers 12–13, 82

British Institute of Learning Disabilities (BILD) 119

Brown, H. 122, 123, 125

Building a Safer NHS for Patients 111

bullying 128

Caldicott Guardians 91

Canada 146, 160

capacity, mental 42, 44–5, 70–1, 114, 123, 129

care contracts 16–17

care in the community 14, 16, 24, 97, 103

care plans 9, 66, 70–1, 75–6, 85–6

for people with long-term health conditions 135

care settings 13–18; abuse in 29–35, **31, 32,** 52, **80–1**; expectations of 34; National Minimum Standards 49–50

Care Standards Act 2000 45–7, **80**; definition of care homes 17; definition of vulnerable adults 23; establishing inspection bodies 55, 59; National Minimum Care Standards 49–50, 61; Protection of Vulnerable Adults list 12,

46–7; speaking out against bad practice 49

carers: abuse by 75–6, 142–5; of people with long-term health conditions 139–41, 142–5; of people with mental health problems 82, 108–10; stress 75, 143–4

Caring for People 118

case conferences 69, 70–1

case records 75, 83–4

child protection education 169

Children Act 2004 88, 93

children, vetting systems for working with 47–8

choice 9, 13–14

classifications of mental disorders 100–1

Clough, R. 34–5, 61

Code of Ethics, BASW 12–13, 82

Codes of Practice: General Social Care Council (GSCC) 10–12, 62, **80**, 82; Mental Capacity Act 2005 44, 45

cognitive behavioural models 76–7

Commission for Health Improvement 10, 112

Commission for Healthcare Audit and Inspection (CHAI) 52, 136, 138

patient safety report 112–13

Commission for Integration and Cohesion 161

Commission for Social Care Inspection (CSCI) 10, 50–1, 52, 55, **56**, 58, 59, 60–1; abuse in care settings in Cornwall 113, 116, 122

Community Care Act 2003 87

Community Care Assessments 8, 9, 18, 66

community-level abuse 149–64; anti-discriminatory practice 153–4; anti-oppressive practice 153–8, 160, 162–3; of asylum seekers and refugee communities 158–64

Community Safety Partnerships/Schemes 152

community work 150–3

complaints 33, 61

Comprehensive Performance Assessments (CPAs) 58–9

confidentiality issues 83, 84, 91

consent, determining 123

context of care, changing 16–17

continual professional development 62–3

contracts, care 16–17

Cornwall, report on learning disability services in 113, 116, 121, 122

Councils with Social Service Responsibilities (CSSRs): commissioning services 8; duties

of 39–40, 68; responses to asylum seekers 161; risk and dangerousness policies and procedures 75; setting up Adult Protection Committees (APCs) 89; *see also* local authorities
Counsel & Care 94
court cases 125, 128–9; Longcare homes 122
criminal justice system 88, 103, 125, 128–9
criminality of abuse 30, 32–3, 38, 125, 126
Crown Courts 129
CSSRs *see* Councils with Social Service Responsibilities
culturagrams 163, **164**
cultural competence 157–8

Data Protection Act 1998 91
dementia care 12, 19, 74, 82
Department of Constitutional Affairs 44, 91
depersonalisation 14, 15
Disability Discrimination Act 1995 138
discriminatory abuse 28, 29, 171; anti-discriminatory versus anti-oppressive practice 153–4; of ethnic groups 162; of people with learning disabilities 120; of people with long-term health conditions 134, 138–9, 145; of people with mental health problems 114; in social care settings 80–3
disease model 99–101
domestic abuse: interventions for **81**; legislation 41–2; moves to institutional care following 29; multi-agency teams for 168; of people with learning disabilities 122; of people with long-term health conditions 141–5, 148
Domestic Violence, Crime and Victims Act 2004 41
domestic violence organisations 90, 141
Domestic Violence Projects 168
Dominelli, L. 156, 161
DSM-IV classification 101

Economic and Social Research Council Violence Research Programme 37–8
education, professional 169
empathy 70, 170
employers: Codes of Practice for 12, **80**; vetting and barring of care staff 46–8
equal opportunities policies 81
ethical practice 49–50, 166
ethnic communities, anti-oppressive practice towards 162–3
ethnicity 151; and mental health 103–4

European Union 148
evidence-based practice 63, 76
evidence, submitting 129

Fair Access to Care Services 14, 40
familial homicide 42
Family Law Act 41
family therapy 168
financial abuse 27; case studies 86, 123–4
France 147
Freedom of Information Act 2000 91

General Social Care Council (GSCC) 55, **56**; Codes of Practice 10–12, 62, **80**, 82
Germany 147
Goffman, E. 14–15, 102

harassment 39, 81, 128
Hayes, D. 159–60, 161
Health Act 1999 9
Health and Social Care Act 2001 87
health care: blurring of boundaries with social care 9, 18, 87; changing role of 9; communications with other agencies 20–1; inter-agency collaboration 87, 90; prioritising adult protection 91; professional education 169
Healthcare Commission report 113, 116, 122
helplines 147
Home Office vulnerable witness survey 2001 129
homophobic abuse 152
hospitals: admissions for long-term health conditions 136; long-stay 35, 97, 117; *see also* psychiatric hospitals
Human Rights Act 1998 91

ICD-10 classification 101
immigration policies 161–2
In Safe Hands 88, 129
independence, promoting 9; case studies 24, 117; in people with learning difficulties 117, 124, 125, 127; in people with long-term health difficulties 133–4
Independent Mental Capacity Advocate (IMCA) 45
information gathering 84–7; from adults with learning disabilities 126–7; life-story approach 127; oral history-taking 126–7; reminiscence work 126
information sharing 91
Inspecting for Better Lives – Delivering Change 60

inspections 35, 50–2, 60–1, 168; *see also* Commission for Social Care Inspection (CSCI)

institutions 13–16; abusive regimes in 27–33, **31, 32**; causes of abuse in 34–5; changes in 16; definitions of 13; depersonalisation in 14, 15; interventions 51–2, **80**, 168; model of 'total' 14–15; moves from domestic abuse to 29; risk factors for abuse in 33–4

inter-agency collaboration 87–94; Adult Protection Committees (APCs) 89–90, 94; for asylum seekers 160; barriers to 90–1, 93; for domestic violence 168; for people with learning disabilities 120–1; strengths of 92–3

International Association of Schools of Social Work 10

International Federation of Social Workers 10

international interventions 146–8

interviews, assessment 73–5, 126–7

Irish community in the UK 151, 161

Italy 147

Jack, R. 12, 13

Japan 147

Johnson, M. 113, 146

Juklestad, O. **32**, 34, 146, 147

Kelly, B. 102, 103

labelling theory 101–2

Lachs, Mark 167

lasting powers of attorney (LPAs) 45

law on abuse 37–53; prevention and protection 39–41; protecting self and others 43–52; protection from others 41–3; race relations 162

learning disabilities 116–30; abuse and 120, 121–8; audits of practice 122; bullying 128; contractual arrangements for care 16; definitions of 118–19; families of people with 128; independence and 117, 124, 125, 127; inter-agency collaboration 120–1; learning daily living skills 127; long-stay hospitals 35, 97, 117; Longcare homes inquiry 122; reports on services 113, 116, 121, 122; social exclusion and 120; sterilisation of women with 127; terminology 118–20; *Valuing People: A New Strategy for Learning Disability for*

the 21st Century 10, 120–1; witnesses in court cases 128–9

Learning Disability Partnership Boards 121

Learning Disability Task Force 121

life-story approach 127

local authorities: care contracts 16–17; development of integrated care services 88, 89; offering choice to individuals 13–14; performance assessments 56–60; providing best value services 58, 59; regulation of social work 56–60; *see also* Councils with Social Service Responsibilities (CSSRs)

Local Authority and Social Services Act 89

Local Government Act 1999 58

long-stay hospitals 37, 97, 117

long-term health conditions 131–47, **137**; abuse and 141–5, 148; adult protection procedures for 142; carers of people with 139–41, 142–5; defining 133–4; demographics of 134; discrimination against people with 134, 138–9, 145; hospital admissions for 136; international interventions for young people with 148; National Service Framework 134–5, 136, 138; patient surveys 128; promoting independence 133–4; service provision for 134–8; social exclusion and 138

Longcare Homes in Buckingham 122

Macpherson Report (1999) 152

Mangelrud Project 146–7

Manthorpe, J. 112, 123, 126

MAPPA (Multi-Agency Public Protection Arrangements) 168

MARAC (Multi-Agency Risk Assessment Conference) 168

Marshall, J. 61

material abuse 27, 132; of people with learning disabilities 123

medical model 99–101

medication abuse 42, 122

mental capacity 42, 44–5, 70–1, 114, 123, 129

Mental Capacity Act 2005 44–5, 72, 114

Mental Deficiency Act 117

mental health 95–115; abuse and 110–15, **115**; adult protection procedures 110, 112, 113; care in the community and 97, 103; carers 108–10; classifications of mental disorders 100–1; defining 97–9; ethnicity and 103–4; labelling theory

101–2; models of 99–106; National
Service Framework 14, 106–7; neurotic
disorder case study 96–7; offending
behaviour and 103; preventing mental ill
health 105–6; safety in mental health
settings 111–13; sexual incidents in
mental health settings 42–3, 111–12;
Sexual Offences Act 2003 and 42–3; social
exclusion of people with mental health
problems 103, 106, 114, 121; strategy and
policy 106–8; terminology 98–9
Mental Health Act 1983 39; under review
43–4, 108
Mental Health Act Commission (MHAC) 10,
52, 112
Mental Health Bill 2006 43–4, 108
Mental Health Foundation 123
Mental Health National Service Framework
14, 106–7
Mental Health Patients in the Community
Act 1995 108
Merton, learning disability services in 116
METIS project 148
Mexico 147
migration patterns in the UK 161–2
Milner, J. 65, 70
models of mental health and illness 99–106
modernising agenda 2, 57, 88, 106
Modernising Mental Health Services 106
Modernising Social Services 40–1, 45, 58
morale of care staff 32, 34, 35, 81
Multi-agency Management Committees
89–90, 94
Multi-Agency Public Protection
Arrangements (MAPPA) 168
Multi-Agency Risk Assessment Conference
(MARAC) 168
multi-agency working 88, 89, 90, 91, 92, 93;
see also partnership working

National Assistance Act 1948 39
National Care Standards Commission 10
National Health Service and Community
Care Act 1990 39–40
National Minimum Standards 49–50, 61
National Occupational Standards for Social
Work 10
National Patient Safety Agency (NPSA)
111–12
National Reporting and Learning System
(NRLS) 111
National Service Frameworks 106; for
long-term health conditions 134–5, 136,
138; for mental health 14, 106–7; for
older people 14, 88
neglect 28, 83; case studies 87, 142–5;
interventions for 168; self-neglect 29
National Health Service and Community
Care Act, 1990 8, 16, 55, 66
NHS Plan 106
No Secrets: abuse in care settings 47, 52;
assessing abuse 68, 69–71, 89; assessing
mental capacity 114; criminality of abuse
30; people with physical health difficulties
141; sexual abuse 123; 'vulnerable adults'
in 24; vulnerable witnesses 129
Norway 146–7
Norwegian Centre on Violence and
Traumatic Stress Studies 147
nursing homes: choosing 14; closure of 51–2,
168; regulatory framework for 50–2; *see
also* institutions

O'Byrne, P. 65, 70
O'Callaghan, A.C. 124, 125
occupational therapists 9, 135
Offences Against the Person Act 1861 39
offending behaviour 103
older people: abuse in mental health settings
112; Action on Elder Abuse 83, 94, 142,
147; developing vulnerability to abuse
132–3; helpline 147; inspection into
services for 60; international interventions
for 146–8; National Service Framework
14, 88; protection procedures for abuse of
167; in service user groups 19; sexual
abuse of 146
oppression *see* anti-oppressive practice
oppression continuum 156–7
oral history-taking 126–7
'othering' process 15, 124, 171
Our Health, Our Care, Our Say 40, 47, 55,
107–8

palliative care 18
Parker, J. **32**, 65, 66, 68, 70, 71, 76, 80, 153,
158, 163, **164**
Parkinson's disease 139
partnership working 87, 88, 93, 94
patient information 83–4, 91
Payne, M. 8, 150
penal institutions 14, 103
Penhale, B. 35, 73, 89, 91, 112, 139
Performance Assessment Framework (PAF)
59–60
Performance Indicators (PIs) 59

performance management 54–64, 55;
    Comprehensive Performance Assessments
    (CPAs) 58–9; critique of 61–2; of
    individual practitioners 62–4; of local
    authorities 56–60; Social Services
    Performance Assessment 59–60; value of
    services 58, 59
'person-first' approach 19, 120
physical abuse 27; of people with learning
    difficulties 122
physical disabilities 138–9; international
    interventions for young people with 148;
    see also long-term health conditions
police: inter-agency collaboration 87;
    involvement in abuse cases 30, 32, 126;
    prioritising adult protection 91
Police Reform Act 2002 87
POVA list (Protection of Vulnerable Adults
    list) 12, 46–7
power and abuse 12, 14
Present State Examination (PSE) 100
Primary Care Teams 9
Primary Care Trusts 9
prisons 14, 103
professional education 169
protection see adult protection procedures
Protection from Harassment Act 1997 39
Protection of Children Act 1999 47
Protection of Vulnerable Adults (POVA) list
    12, 46–7
psychiatric assessment 44, 99–101
psychiatric hospitals 16, 102, 103; abuse in
    110; common views of 97; facilities in
    112
psychological abuse 27
psychological factors for mental health
    problems 104
Public Concern at Work 83, 94
Public Interest Disclosure Act 1998 49, 80

quality assurance 62–3

racism: attitudes to people with mental health
    problems 103–4; Community Safety
    Partnerships 152; in the implementation
    of the Mental Health Act 1983 44;
    legislation outlawing 162
racist abuse 28, 29
record keeping 75, 83–4
refugee communities 158–64
refuges for women 148
Registered Homes Act 1984 16, 50–2, 55, 80
registration 50–2, 87

regulation of social work and social services
    56–64; critique of 61
rehabilitation services 136, 138
relatives, abuse by 81
reminiscence work 126
residential care homes: case study of neglect
    87; choice of 13–14; closure of 51–2, 168;
    regulatory framework for 50–2; small 16,
    50; see also institutions
respite care 16, 135
risk assessment 73–5, 85, 168
risk factors for abuse in institutions 33–4
risks, the right to take 71–2
Rowan Ward inquiry 112
Rowe, Gordon 122
Royal Commission 1957 118

Safeguarding Adults 50
Safeguarding Boards 89–90, 94
Safeguarding Vulnerable Groups Act 2006
    47, 48
safety: community schemes 152; issues in
    assessment interviews 73–4; in mental
    health settings 111–13
Sainsbury Centre for Mental Health 112
schizophrenia 102–3
Scotland: legislation in 38–9, 129;
    'Supporting Police, Protecting
    Communities' (2005) 152
self-neglect 29
sensory impairments 134
service user groups 1–2, 18–21
sexual abuse 27, 129, 148; case studies 32–3,
    128; in mental health settings 111–12; of
    older people 146; of people with learning
    difficulties 122–3
Sexual Offences Act 2003 42–3, 88
Single Assessment Process 88–9
skills for social care workers 76–7
Smale, G. 65, 70
social care practitioners: abuse by 12, 27–33,
    34–5, 80; abuse of 12, 30; changing role
    of 19; code of ethics 12–13, 82; code of
    practice 10–12, 62, 82; communication
    problems between agencies 20–1;
    evidence-based practice 63, 76;
    involvement in community protection
    plans 152–3; performance management
    62–4; professional education 169; status
    and morale 32, 34, 35, 81; supervision of
    81–2, 169–70; supporting people with
    learning difficulties 120, 122–3;
    supporting people with long-term health

conditions 135, 136, 137; supporting witnesses in court cases 128–9; theory and skills for 76–7; training and development 12, 62–3, 81, 84; vetting and barring systems 46–8; whistle blowing 49, **80**, 83, 94; *see also* social workers
social constructionism 25–6
social exclusion 171; of people with learning disabilities 120; of people with mental health problems 103, 106, 114, 121; of people with physical disabilities 138
social factors for mental health problems 104, 105–6
social model: of disability 138; of mental health 99, 101–4
social need 66–7, 159
Social Services Performance Assessment 59–60
social work 8–13; blurring of boundaries with health care 9, 18, 87; concerns over quality 61; definition 10; modernising agenda 2, 57, 88, 106; regulation of 56–64; 'visibility' in 55, **56**
social workers: changing role of 18; code of ethics 12–13, 82; code of practice 10–12, 62, 82; communications with other agencies 20–1, 44; community 156–7; continual professional development 62–3; professional education 169; review under the Mental Health Act 1983 43–4; specializing in mental health 99, 105, 115; supervision and support for 169–70; theory and skills 76–7; working with asylum seekers 159–63; *see also* social care practitioners
societal abuse *see* discriminatory abuse
specialist equipment 133–4
Standards on Adult Protection 50
status of care staff 32, 34, 35, 81
Strategy Meetings 69–70
stress: carers' 75, 143–4; links to abuse 63; links to mental health problems 105
stroke patients 20, 134, 136, 138, 139
'structural violence' 103
supervision of social care practitioners 81–2, 169–70
'Supporting Police, Protecting Communities' (2005) 152
Sutton, learning disability services in 116

theory for social care workers 76–7
Thompson, N. 123, 153–4, 155; PCS interactive model of oppression 155
training: in adult protection procedures 12, 62–3, 84, 122–3; case study 57; in inclusive policies 81; multi-agency strategy 168–9
transphobic abuse 152
traveller communities 158
Turk, V. 122, 123

Ulleval project 146–7
United States 146, 147–8, 167

Valuing People: A New Strategy for Learning Disability for the 21st Century 10, 120–1
vetting systems 46–8
violence: interventions for 168; legislation on protection from 38; in mental health settings 112; recording incidents of 75; *see also* domestic abuse
visibility in social care practices 55, **56**
vulnerable adults: citizenship rights of 49; defining 23–4; involving 65–6, 70, 73–4; right to take risks 71–2; as service user groups 18–21
vulnerable witnesses 128–9
Vulnerable Witnesses (Scotland) Act 2004 129

Wales: Adult Protection Committees (APCs) 89; *In Safe Hands* 88, 129
welfare: argument of abuse 30, 32, 38, 125; for asylum seekers 159–60
whistle blowing 49, **80**, 83, 94
White Papers: *Better Services for the Mentally Handicapped* 118, 120; *Caring for People* 118; Local Government (2006) 88; *Modernising Social Services* 40–1, 45, 58; *Our Health, Our Care, Our Say* 40, 47, 55, 107–8; *Valuing People: A New Strategy for Learning Disability for the 21st Century* 10, 120–1
Who Decides? 24
witnesses in court cases 128–9
World Health Organization (WHO) 97

Youth Justice and Criminal Evidence Act 1999 129

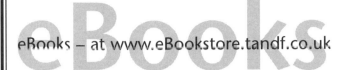